Social Foundations of Behavior for the Health Sciences

Ginny Garcia-Alexander • Hyeyoung Woo
Matthew J. Carlson

Social Foundations of Behavior for the Health Sciences

Springer

Ginny Garcia-Alexander
Department of Sociology
Portland State University
Portland, Oregon, USA

Hyeyoung Woo
Department of Sociology
Portland State University
Portland, Oregon, USA

Matthew J. Carlson
Department of Sociology
Portland State University
Portland, Oregon, USA

ISBN 978-3-319-64948-1 ISBN 978-3-319-64950-4 (eBook)
DOI 10.1007/978-3-319-64950-4

Library of Congress Control Number: 2017949870

Printed on acid-free paper

This Springer imprint is published by Springer Nature
The registered company is Springer International Publishing AG
The registered company address is: Gewerbestrasse 11, 6330 Cham, Switzerland

To Tyler, David, and Kristin, for their endless support.

Preface

This book provides students in the health sciences with a foundation in sociology along with an understanding of social factors and processes and their impacts on health. It is designed to develop the necessary knowledge and background required by the newly added section of the medical college entrance exam, "Psychological, Social, and Biological Foundations of Behavior". It reviews the fundamental concepts of an introductory sociology text with attention to how such concepts connect to health at multiple levels. Thus, each chapter is designed in accordance with the related content on the exam and offers a general overview of the major sociological concepts, concrete examples of how concepts can be applied in a health setting, key terms and definitions, activities and research examples (that can be utilized in the classroom or individually), example study questions, and recommended external links and resources. As an additional bonus, it includes the specific content coverage from the exam in each chapter with references to the specific content categories and what they test.

Extended Table of Contents and Descriptions

Chapter 1
Introduction to Sociology and Socio-Cultural Impacts on Health

Objectives

- Recognize importance of socio-cultural impacts on health
- Define social determinants of health
- Introduce and define basic concepts in sociology and major theoretical perspectives

Newly Added Foundational Concepts from Exam

The changes to the 2015 exam include new sections on Psychological, Social and Biological Foundations of Behavior. This section will test examinees' knowledge and use of the concepts in psychology, sociology, biology, research methods, and statistics that provide a solid foundation for learning about the behavioral and socio-cultural determinants of health and health outcomes in medical school. Understanding the behavioral and socio-cultural determinants of health is important to the study of medicine. You will be tested on your knowledge of the ways in which psychological, social, and biological factors influence perceptions and reactions to the world; behavior, and behavior change; what people think about themselves and others; the cultural and social differences that influence well-being; and the relationships between social stratification, access to resources, and well-being.

The relevance of social scientific research to medical practice is now recognized, and per the Association of American Medical Colleges recommendations are best understood through the key themes of: 1) research approaches that are theory driven and based on behavioral and social perspectives, 2) a vantage point that considers the source of individual variation, and 3) emphasizes variation across sociodemographic factors and their sources (AAMC 2011). Throughout this text, students will find explicit connections to the

(continued)

G. Garcia-Alexander et al., *Social Foundations of Behavior for the Health Sciences*,
DOI 10.1007/978-3-319-64950-4_1

learning modules found in the exam study guide and a wealth of examples that apply the concepts described in a health setting. This text further provides a basic understanding of *sociological* concepts, with special attention to the concepts emphasized in the exam.

Foundational Concepts contained in this chapter include: **Concept 7** (Psychological, socio-cultural, and biological factors influence behavior and behavior change) and **Concept 9** (Cultural and social differences influence well-being).

1.1 Socio-cultural Impacts on Health

It has come to be well-recognized that there is a strong and enduring link between various social factors and characteristics (including such things as race/ethnicity, poverty status, insurance coverage, etc.) and health behaviors, status, and outcomes. These relationships are complex and impact health both directly and indirectly. For example, the direct impact of race/ethnicity is evidenced in poorer infant mortality outcomes among African American women. In other words, it has long been observed that black infants die at rates more than double that of non-Hispanic white infants (Frieden 2013). Indirectly, racial/ethnic differences in quality of- and access to- care have also been observed. For example, an increasing number of studies have shown that racial and ethnic minorities experience barriers to accessing care, even after controlling for insurance coverage and income (IOM 2003). It is also more difficult to obtain quality care for some groups. Thus, we observe differences in prescribing behaviors, recommendations for procedures, and so on. Such differences may stem from stereotyping, time pressures, language barriers, or other factors tied to the clinical encounter. Importantly, these differences in access and quality exert their own harmful impacts on health status. While the exact causes of these discrepancies remain unclear, their presence is undeniable, and moving toward ***health equity*** has become an important goal in the United States. In fact, the Healthy People 2020 goals are expressly committed to improving health outcomes and increasing health equity. In order to achieve these goals, it is necessary for those in health-related fields to recognize the impacts of social factors on health.

Research that connects social factors to health has largely come from the work of researchers in fields including sociology, psychology, economics, and public health, to name a few. Scholars in these disciplines have successfully confirmed the importance of understanding how health is impacted in ways that are not purely biological or genetic in nature. They have further helped us to understand how social inequities lead to *avoidable* gaps in health. Thus, this book will describe and introduce the different social factors that are connected to health, provide various examples of how these factors impact health-related outcomes, and offer resources and tools for developing skills in cultural competency. As health professionals, it is necessary to acknowledge and understand the role of social factors in order to provide an adequate level of care in health settings.

In this introductory chapter, we describe the key terms and concepts necessary to developing competence in the social foundations of health status and behaviors. In addition, we will review some of the basic terminology and core concepts in sociology as it provides the tools to understand how social structures and processes influence our lives. These concepts help form the foundation for developing competency in the *Psychological, Social, and Biological Foundation of Behavior* section, described in AAMC's 2015 study guide. Specific topics in this chapter and throughout the book connect directly to specific foundational concepts and content categories. Concepts that link directly to content categories are identified with information on where they may be found in the newly developed section of the exam.

Key Terms

Social determinants of health: the economic and social conditions that influence individual and group differences in health status. "Social determinants of health reflect the social factors and physical conditions of the environment in which people are born, live, learn, play, work, and age. Also known as social and physical determinants of health, they impact a wide range of health, functioning, and quality-of-life outcomes." (Healthy People 2020) http://www.healthypeople.gov/2020/about/foundation-health-measures/Determinants-of-Health

- Examples of social determinants:
  - Resource availability (job and education opportunities, access to healthy food, presence of medical providers or hospitals with NIC facilities)
  - Social norms and attitudes *see definitions below and chapter on race/ethnicity for more information on the role of discrimination to health outcomes
  - Exposure to crime and neighborhood disorder
  - Social support and social isolation
  - Exposure to mass media and emerging technologies
  - Socioeconomic conditions (e.g. concentrated poverty)
  - Mode of transportation and commute time
  - Exposure to environmental toxins
  - Public safety
  - Residential segregation

- Upstream factors (upstream social determinants): "fundamental causes that set in motion causal pathways leading to (often temporally and spatially distant) health effects through downstream factors" (Braveman et al. 2011)
- Downstream factors (downstream social determinants): "factors that are temporally and spatially close to health effects (and hence relatively apparent), but are influenced by upstream factors" (Braveman et al. 2011)

In epidemiology and public health, a metaphor is often used to explain the upstream/downstream factors and how they impact health. In this metaphor a river represents the flow, or pathways, through which various factors impact health. If there is a factory located upstream that pollutes the river with toxic chemicals and a population of individuals who live downstream, the various responses to that toxic runoff may be thought of as upstream or downstream. If the response is to filter the contaminated water, that's a downstream response since it is occurring at the level of the individual (and further places the burden on the individual for making a change or correcting the issue). More downstream recommendations might include

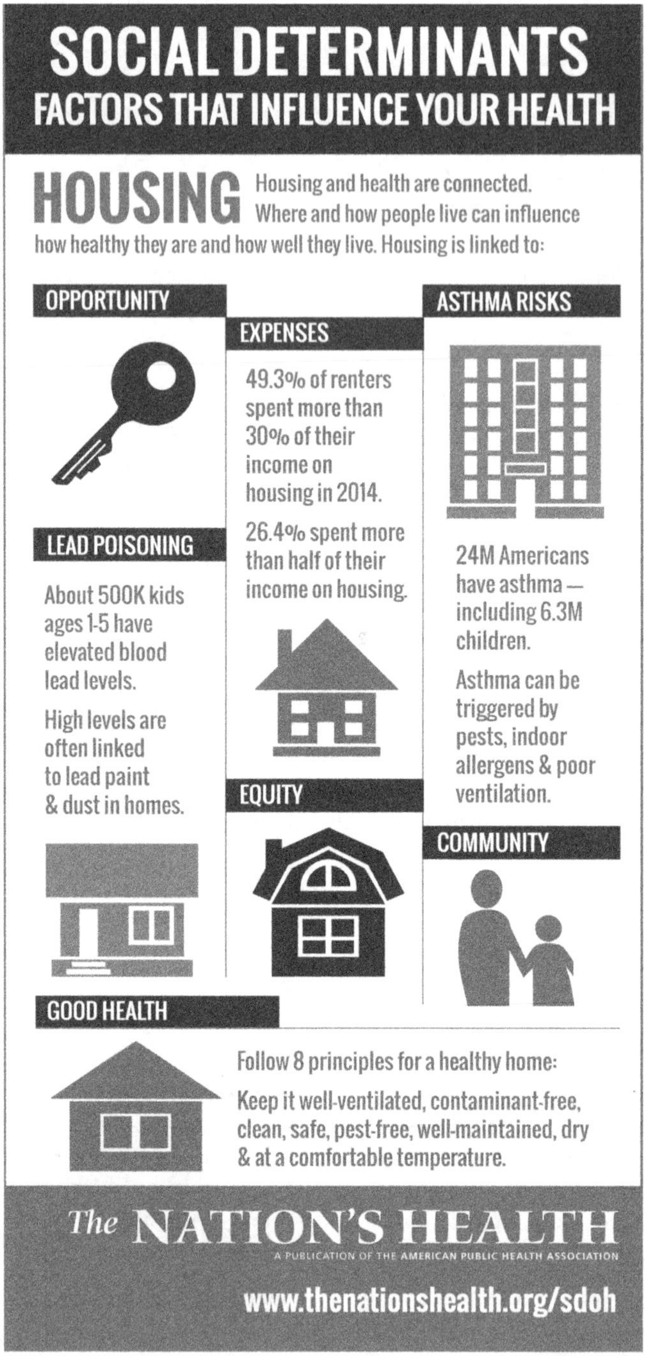

Social determinants of health (Source: The Nation's Health Series: Social Determinants of Health, American Public Health Association. http://thenationshealth.aphapublications.org/site/misc/socialdeterminants.xhtml)

For more information, visit https://students-residents.aamc.org/applying-medical-school/article/whats-mcat-exam/

telling people to move away from the most polluted areas or recommending the purchase of bottled water for drinking. One can easily imagine how these remedies might be easier for those with more resources. If, however the response is to make it illegal to dump toxic chemicals into the river, that's an upstream response that focuses on the true source of what's producing harmful influences on health.

Health Equity: (as defined by Healthy People 2020) is the "attainment of the highest level of health for all people. Achieving health equity requires valuing everyone equally with focused and ongoing societal efforts to address avoidable inequalities historical and contemporary injusticesand the elimination of health and health care disparities."

Health Disparity: as defined by Healthy People 2020, is "a particular type of health difference that is closely linked with social, economic, and/or environmental disadvantage. Health disparities adversely affect groups of people who have systematically experienced greater obstacles to health based on their racial or ethnic group; religion; socioeconomic status; gender; age; mental health; cognitive, sensory, or physical disability; sexual orientation or gender identity; geographic location; or other characteristics historically linked to discrimination or exclusion."

1.2 A General Introduction to Sociology

What is sociology? **Sociology** is the study of social life. It applies a scientific approach to the identification and examination of patterns of human behavior. It explores group processes and how they affect (and are affected by) **social structures** and **institutions**. Formally, **social structures** are organized patterns of social relationships and institutions that constitute society. They can be thought of as the framework of society, which works to guide our behavior and is in turn, shaped by human responses to the structure. **Social institutions** are established and organized systems of social behavior with a specified purpose, e.g. the family, marriage, education. These institutions exist to ensure the overall welfare of society by socializing new members, maintaining stability and existence, and providing members with a sense of purpose.

One of the key assumptions of sociology is that all human behavior has a social context. That means that we recognize that we are individuals who are capable of making decisions based on free will, but the choices we make are guided and shaped by social forces. For example, a person might choose to become a doctor and actively pursue that goal. But, the decision was likely influenced by how the person was raised, who they were raised by, where they grew up, and so on. In addition, the ability to achieve that goal is also influenced by the quality of education they have access to, their personal characteristics, and their socioeconomic position, among other things. Sociologists further recognize that there is a hierarchy to the social system that influences our access to a number of social institutions. This hierarchy is referred to as **social stratification**. As mentioned above, a person's position in the social system can have very real and measureable impacts on their health.

Sociology developed as a discipline during the Enlightenment period, also known as the Age of Reason. This occurred during the eighteenth century and signified a time in human history when reason and rationality were emphasized, and scientific explanations were used to understand the laws of collective social life. Much like the scientific method was applied in the natural sciences; the earliest sociologists were committed to discovering the laws of human and social behavior (a way of thinking known as positivism) and using them to help solve society's problems. For example, the French philosopher Auguste Comte (1798–1857) advocated for the study of human society in a highly scientific manner. Following his lead, Emile Durkheim (1858–1917) contributed a great deal to the influence of sociology as a discipline and to developing a science of society. He argued that a clear set of principles, or **theories** of social behavior, needed to be developed so that they could be rigorously tested using scientific methods (Fig. 1.1).

Theory (def.): A set of principles and propositions that explains the relationships between social phenomena. Theories provide abstract, but testable explanations of observable phenomena.

An important theoretical perspective developed by Emile Durkheim is **functionalism**. This particular theory likens social structures and their mechanisms to those of a biological organism. It argues that much like the brain, heart, and various other organs must work together (and perform specific functions) to maintain equilibrium within the body, so too must the various social institutions work together to maintain society. He argued that societies were based on established rules and practices that were passed down through various social institutions like the family or educational system. These institutions take on different forms and serve various necessary functions which keep society in balance. Functionalists believe that social arrangements can be understood in terms of the functions they serve. For example, a functionalist

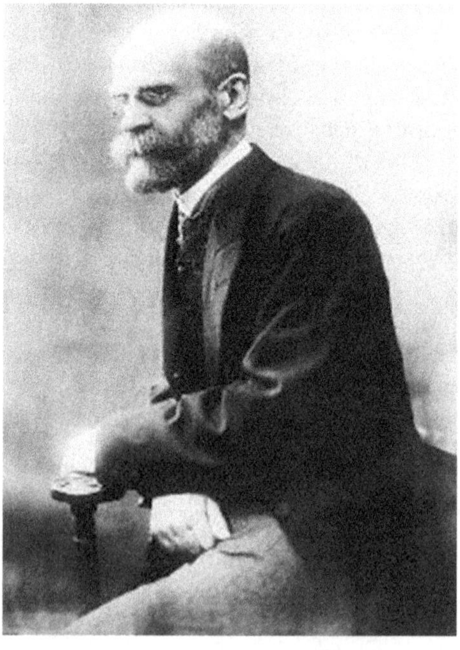

Fig. 1.1 Emile Durkheim (Photo Credit: PD-1923)

perspective on the presence of poverty would argue that it creates a class a class of individuals who are willing to take undesirable jobs, it generates job opportunities for those that serve the poor, and it creates motivation to succeed or differentiate oneself from those in poverty. Generally, if society is in balance, i.e. performing in a way that benefits the system, individuals are well-integrated, and collectively healthy and happy. Durkheim referred to an integrated system as *organic* or *social solidarity.*

In an important study that helped to launch the discipline of sociology, Durkheim systematically tracked and described how social factors influence suicide *(Suicide: A Study in Sociology* (1897)*)*, something that is easily thought of as an individual act. Most importantly, it allowed him to show that there were distinct patterns to human behavior and that suicide had social roots by linking the characteristics of various groups/societies to their rates of suicide. Specifically, he observed that rates of suicide were highly stable from year to year on the basis of characteristics including religion, marital status, and socioeconomic background. For example, he observed that suicide was more common in non-married persons compared to those who were married. He further observed that the rates were highly variable from place to place, i.e. small, close-knit societies versus modern, industrialized societies. He explained these differences with the concept of social integration and suggested that in modern society individuals were less integrated (or lacked moral regulation) while they were more socially integrated in traditional societies. In other words, the more strongly one was connected with or integrated in society, the lower their likelihood of suicide. He further introduced the concept of *anomie*, which refers to a feeling of aimlessness (a lack of social norms tied to weakened social attachments present in modern society).

Another major theorist who contributed greatly to the development of the discipline and **conflict theory** was Karl Marx (1818–1883). In contrast to Durkheim, who focused on social integration, Marx concentrated on class differences. He argued that society was inherently unequal and that different groups possessed varying amounts of power, prestige, and wealth. These inherent inequalities produce conflicts of interest between the 'haves' versus the 'have-nots.' Marx further believed that the injustices and inequalities present in a capitalist system would lead to the breakdown of capitalist societies (Appelrouth and Edles 2012). In one of his most famous essays, *The Communist Manifesto* (Marx and Engels [1846] 1977), he developed **conflict theory** which focuses on the imbalance of power between those groups with greater advantages relative to those who are disadvantaged. Formally, he distinguished groups in relation to the means of production and identified the bourgeoisie as the owners of capital (those with power), and the proletariat as the property-less wage earners (with little access to power). The theory further posits that inequality is perpetuated by the established rules and systems put into place by those in power to ensure they remain in power. Going back to the poverty example, a conflict theorist would focus on who's in power and how various social structures work to produce an unequal system that generates poverty for specific groups. Thus, a conflict theorist might emphasize the importance of an unequal educational system, which provides unfair advantages to some while restricting access and opportunities for others (Fig. 1.2).

A final theorist who had an important impact on the discipline and together with Durkheim and Marx, is considered to be one of the classic founders of sociology, is Max Weber (1864–1920). His work was influenced by Marx, though he argued that there was more to conflict than economic standings alone. Thus, he argued that

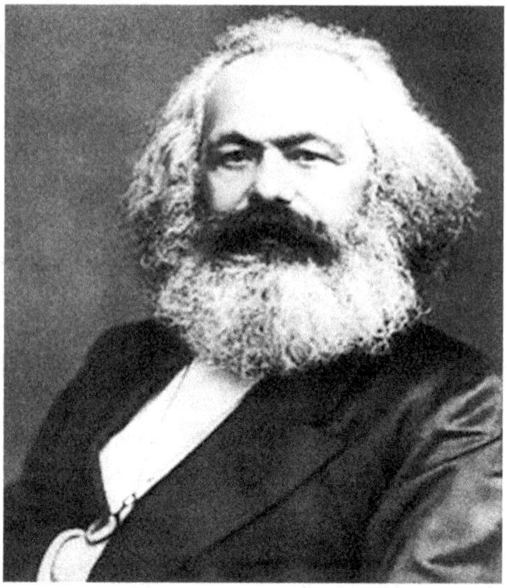

Fig. 1.2 Karl Marx (Photo Credit: PD-1923)

one's life chances were influenced by prestige and political influence in addition to their material wealth (a major contribution was *Economy and Society* (1925)). Much of Weber's work focused on the impact of ideas and values, and how modern society was characterized by rationalization. In one of his most famous works, *The Protestant Ethic and the Spirit of Capitalism* (1904), he argued that the properties of Protestantism/Christianity allowed capitalism to take root and become the dominant mode of production.

Taken together, these theorists had a tremendous impact on the discipline. While their orientations to the study of society were quite different, they were each motivated by historical circumstances that produced rapid and dramatic shifts in society. These changes are referred to as modernity, a term which encompasses the concepts of: capitalism, mass production, industrialization, densely populated urban centers, western dominance, and secularization (Jones et al. 2011). These characteristics fundamentally changed the nature of society and social interaction. The theoretical perspectives (functionalism and conflict theory) developed by these figures to explain the tenets of modern society can be thought of as macro-theories. Formally, **macro-sociological** perspectives are those that focus on the study of large-scale social systems (Giddens et al. 2014). These types of theories consider the impacts of broader social forces, i.e. social structures, on social behavior.

In contrast to macro-sociological perspectives, **micro-** perspectives focus on the everyday details of face-to-face interaction. Micro-theories take a close-up view of society by examining how everyday interactions produce social reality. They are based on the assumption that humans take a very active and creative role in shaping society. An important micro-sociological theory that Herbert Blumer (1900–1987) developed based on the work of George Herbert Mead (1863–1931) was **symbolic interaction**. As the title indicates, this theory focuses on the interaction of humans via the use of symbols. Formally, a symbol is an item which represents something. For example, a cross represents Christianity. Language is also a symbol, and perhaps society's most important one, which is used to communicate meaning. A key element of this theory is meaningful **social interaction**, which refers to a two-way process in which meaning is communicated through language (or other forms of communication) and is interpreted. Thus, when we interact with others, we communicate with them, gauge their reactions to our communications and alter our behavior in accordance with our interpretation of the effects of the communication. For example, when we visit a doctor's office for the first time, we may attempt to explain in great detail the nature of our illness. If however, the doctor interrupts or shifts their attention to some other task, we may cut short our explanation and assume the doctor is too busy to listen to our explanation. Alternately, if the doctor nods and listens intently, we may feel encouraged to continue explaining. Accordingly, we have ascribed meaning to the doctor's reactions and the nature of the situation shifted to match that understanding.

Social Construction is another micro- perspective developed by sociologists. The concept was introduced by Peter Berger and Thomas Luckmann in, *The Social Construction of Reality* (1966). It refers to the idea that as a society, we develop a reality that is based on shared agreement. More generally, they viewed society as a "subjective reality." In other words, our reality is determined by the subjective meanings we attach to various situations. Much of the contemporary work in this area focuses on gender issues, and comes to us from Judith Butler, who explores the importance of social meaning in constructing gender identities. In sociology, we differentiate between the term sex, which refers to biological identity, and gender, which refers to the social meanings associated with each sex. Thus, the *social construction of gender* refers to the idea that there is no objective definition of gender. Instead we construct its meaning in accordance with our views on masculinity and femininity, and these views and perceptions are passed on through the socialization process. Thus, Butler and other proponents of this theory argue that there are no real biological bases for sex differences – gender identity comes from perceived differences based on sex.

Health Example: A prime example of the social construction of reality and how a subjective reality may become real in its consequences relates to the health field. A number of researchers in the field of sociology have examined the health-related consequences of perceived discrimination in the health setting. What they have been able to illustrate successfully is that when individuals perceive discrimination by a health professional, it can result in a host of negative outcomes. It may lead to an avoidance of care or treatment-seeking, or a greater tendency to engage in negative coping mechanisms. It can also have a negative impact on health itself. As an example, researchers have shown that the stress produced by exposure to discrimination and racism results in poorer health outcomes. For a very good review of the sociological contributions to the study of racial and ethnic disparities in health see the article mentioned in the *Resources, Links, and Recommended Readings* section entitled, "Understanding Racial-Ethnic Disparities in Health: Sociological Contributions".

1.3 The Development of Sociology in the United States

The development of American sociology has largely been attributed to sociologists at the University of Chicago (commonly referred to as the Chicago school). However, American sociology evolved during a period of great racial conflict. As such, the scholars of the day (Robert Ezra Park, Ernest Burgess, Albion Small) were not immune to scientific racism and perpetuated racial inequities by ignoring or appropriating the work of black sociologists. Many of their views reflected an unquestioning belief in white supremacy. In some cases, their assertions and findings were overtly racist. For example, Robert Ezra Park, who is largely considered to be one of the most important American sociologists, and Ernest Burgess published their support for eugenics (the practice of selective breeding) in the first American sociology textbook, *Introduction to the Science of Sociology* (1921).

Contemporary scholars are increasingly challenging the idea that the Chicago school was the birthplace of American sociology and calling for attention to the contributions of scholars of color that have long been neglected. They contest the primacy of the Chicago school and instead suggest that the first scientific school of sociology, the DuBois-Atlanta school, was developed in the 1890s at Atlanta University by W.E.B. DuBois (1868–1963) (Morris 2015). DuBois created a sociological laboratory devoted to systematically and empirically studying the causes of racial inequality. It was within this context that the first community studies and empirically derived sociological theories were developed in the U.S. (Morris 2015). DuBois made invaluable contributions to the field of sociology including *The Philadelphia Negro* (1899), *The Souls of Black Folk* (1903), and *Black Reconstruction* (1935). In *The Philadelphia Negro,* he systematically examined the social and living conditions of African Americans by carrying out 5000 surveys and interviews. The Souls of Black Folk is now thought of as one of the most important books written on race in the U.S., within which DuBois developed the notion of the social construction of race. The book received high praise from Max Weber himself, who argued it should be translated to German. DuBois was the first to offer insight on racial consciousness and even discussed the role of stereotypes in *The Souls of White Folk* (1920). Other notable scholars of color include Oliver C. Cox, E. Franklin Frazier, and Charles Johnson. *The Scholar Denied* (2015) (listed in the *Resources, Links, and Recommended Readings* section) provides a thorough and revelatory discussion of the contributions made by black scholars in sociology, and further argues that an entire generation of black scholars has been removed from sociological history (Monroe Work, R.R. Wright, Jr., and George Edmund Haynes) (Fig. 1.3).

The contributions of women have also been neglected in discussions of the development of sociology as a discipline. As an example, Harriet Martineau (1802–1876) was responsible for translating and condensing the work of Auguste Comte (mentioned earlier for coining the term sociology), thus making his work available to English-speakers. She is commonly thought of as the first female sociologist, and her work is all the more impressive given that she conducted a masterful study of American life (*Society in America*) quite a few years before many of those who have been credited with this endeavor. Anna Julia Cooper (1858–1964) offered the first social theory of women of color in, *A Voice from the South by a Black Woman of the*

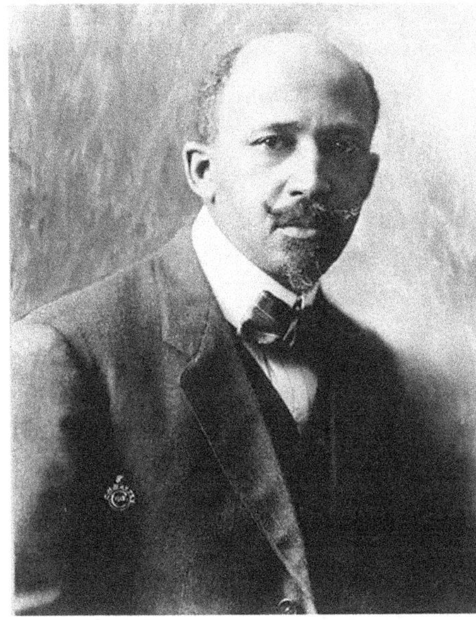

Fig. 1.3 W.E.B. DuBois (Photo credit: PD-1923)

South (1892). Ida B. Wells (1862–1931) is considered one of the earliest contributors to feminist thought. She wrote passionately on her opposition to white violence and lynching, and was a founder of the NAACP (see more on her in the link provided in the *Resources, Links, and Recommended Readings* section).

1.4 The Sociological Imagination

Thinking sociologically involves the ability to see the links between the experiences of individuals and the larger social forces that shape those experiences. The term, **sociological imagination**, was coined by C. Wright Mills and refers to the ability to see those links. Sociologists apply the sociological imagination to the development of sociological questions and theories. C. Wright Mills discussed a series of questions that are relevant in this context. These include: "(1) What is the structure of this particular society as a whole?. (2) Where does this society stand in human history?. (3) What varieties of men and women now prevail in this society and in this period?" (C. Wright Mills 1959). In addition, he developed the terms, troubles and issues, to distinguish incidents that impact an individual versus those that are broader in nature. He argued that troubles were those things that immediately impacted the individual. On the other hand, issues are those that are larger than the individual and constitute a public matter. For example, if an individual struggles with their weight and is overweight or obese, that would be classified as a trouble. Thinking sociologically about overweight and obesity involves the ability to recognize that this is an issue that impacts over two-thirds of Americans and is heavily impacted by such things as available food choices, food policies, and health-related behaviors, among others. Sociology shows us the need to look beyond the surface of people's circumstances and actions, to the impact of social forces on the issue.

Key Terms and Definitions

- **Sociology**: A social science used to understand the patterns of human behavior in society.
- **Sociological Imagination**: a term coined by C. Wright Mills which describes the ability to see the link between incidents in the lives of individuals and large social forces (involves the ability to differentiate between troubles and issues).
- **Macro-sociology** (Content Category 9A): seeks to understand and explain large-scale social systems; addresses comparisons among larger groups (e.g. states)
- **Micro-sociology** (Content Category 9A): focuses on the smallest, most immediately visible aspects of social life; examines interactions among individuals and small groups
- **Social structure**: any group characteristic; they influence our behavior in much the same way physical structures channel our movements
- **Social institutions**: Relatively permanent patterns or clusters of specialized roles, groups, organizations, customs, and activities devoted to meeting fundamental social needs; a weave of behaviors, norms, and values
- **Social interaction**: An exchange between two or more people that is given meaning.
- **Social Norms** (Content Category 7B): The principles or rules of social life that people are expected to observe "normal behavior"; Most all of us want to be seen as normal so we adjust our behavior to be perceived as such
- **Diversity**: a characteristic of a society which has a variety thought, religion, national origin, race, sexual orientation, etc. In the U.S., our social policies generally support the idea that differences should be tolerated and respected. A number of policies have been enacted to combat racism, prevent unfair treatment, protect various minority groups, and ensure equal access to opportunities.
- **Stratification** (Content Category 10A): Relatively fixed hierarchical arrangements in society by which groups have difference access to resources, power, and perceived social worth.
- **Theory** (Content Category 9A): an abstract statement that explains why and how certain things happen or are as they are; provides abstract but testable explanations of observable phenomena
- **Research** (Content Category 9A): making appropriate empirical observations or measurements (in an effort to test theories); involves data collection and data analysis
- **Sociological Theories** (Content Category 9A)
  - **Conflict Theory**: a macro-sociological theory, society is inherently unequal due to a capitalist system which advantages the owning class over the working class
    - Perspective on health: conflict theory focuses on how political and economic structures generate inequality and conflict, which in turn lead to deeply ingrained differences in access to health care and health outcomes among various subgroups

- **Functionalism**: a macro-sociological theory, society is made up of various social structures that work together, or serve a specific function, to ensure equilibrium in society
  - Perspective on health: illness is a form of deviance that disturbs social function, i.e. a sick person is not a contributing member of society. It is the role of the medical profession to address this deviance and impose sanctions
  - **The sick role**: Illness is a social role that carries specific expectations and obligations. When a person experiences illness they are not subject to typical social roles and instead substitute the new sick role. Because it prevents members from contributing to the overall function of society, it is inherently dysfunctional.
- **Symbolic Interaction**: a micro-sociological theory; focuses on subjective meanings and the use of symbols in everyday patterns of interaction
  - Perspective on health: It is the perception and interpretation of strain or stress that leads to real consequences. Thus, if a person perceives/interprets an interaction as stressful or unpleasant (whether real or imagined), it can lead to a real stress response that may lead to disease through wear on the body.
- **Social Constructionism**: The perception of what is real is determined by the subjective meanings we attribute to an experience
  - Perspective on health: race, is a primarily socially constructed category, which does not generate biologically based differences in health outcomes. Racial/ethnic disparities in health outcomes are the product of shared agreement/belief in racial/ethnic differences that translate into differences in access to and quality of care.

Activities and Research Examples

- **Activity 1: the sociological imagination > ask students to brainstorm medical concepts (ex. visiting the doctor's office, women's health, chronic illness, etc.)**

  Deploy the *sociological imagination* on the following. You may want to consider for instance, those social relations and wider social processes and interconnections informing each, or perhaps the ways in which each may involve different claims to social status and distinction. Additionally, you may want to consider their ritual, spatial, and/or temporal features. Remember there are no right answers – only more or less creative attempts at interpretation and recovery of the changing nature of the social.
- **Activity 2: Medicine as an Institution**

  Institutions serve a number of purposes including: 1) socialization of new members, 2) production and distribution of goods and services, 3) replacement of membership, 4) maintain stability and existence of society, and 5) provide a sense of purpose. Consider the needs that our medical system meets, how it functions, modes of access, norms of operation, etc.

- **Research Example 1: Online Interaction and the Institution of Medicine**
  An increasing number of sites/services are now offering "on-demand" medicine that provides access to a physician via app, subscription, etc. Identify such a site and detail how one gets access, what services are offered, etc.
  Next, consider how this may fundamentally change the nature of the patient provider relationship. Is this increasing access to health care for all? What the benefits and disadvantages? Is there an impact on quality of care?
- **Research Example 2: Diverse Needs in the Health Care Setting**
  Our society is increasingly diverse and cultural differences have been shown to impact delivery of health care and health outcomes. Describe the current set of standards for addressing a diverse population. What areas need improvement? How will this potentially affect you in the future?

Study Questions

1. Describe the major elements of conflict theory, functionalism, symbolic interactionism, and social constructionism.

***Example Exam Question:** "Anxious about a nagging illness, a patient feels ignored by a doctor who is struggling to catch up with patient examinations on a very busy day. Conversely, the doctor misinterprets the discomfort and agitation of the patient as hostility. This scenario is most closely related to which paradigm?

A. Functionalism.
B. Conflict Theory.
C. Symbolic Interactionism.
D. Social Constructionism." (AAMC 2012: 131)

*For more information, visit https://students-residents.aamc.org/applying-medical-school/article/whats-mcat-exam/

Resources, Links, and Recommended Readings

Recommended Readings on the Development of Sociology and Race-Related Issues.

Morris, Aldon. (2015). *The Scholar Denied: W.E.B. DuBois and the Birth of Modern Sociology*. Oakland: University of California Press.
Williams, David R., & Michelle Sternthal. (2010). Understanding racial-ethnic disparities in health: Sociological contributions. *Journal of Health and Social Behavior*, 51(S): S15–S27.
Zuberi, Tukufu, & Eduardo Bonilla-Silva. (2008). *White Logic, White Methods: Racism and Methodology*. Lanham: Rowman & Littlefield Publishers.

Boundless Sociology: A free textbook resource developed by a community of educators that provides access to online content and study materials. https://boundless.com/sociology

Cultural Competency Training: Think Cultural Health is a free resource available to health professionals to help promote culturally and linguistically appropriate services. The following link provides access to a series of courses and e-learning programs for those employed in health-related positions. https://www.thinkculturalhealth.hhs.gov/Content/ContinuingEd.asp

Healthy People 2020: A set of objectives developed every 10 years that are aimed at improving the health of all Americans. Link provides access to the list of objectives and an interactive data tool that allows users to examine health outcomes. https://www.healthypeople.gov/

National Center for Health Statistics (NCHS): the nation's principal health agency, which collects and publishes data, and makes health-related recommendations. https://www.cdc.gov/nchs/index.htm

The Rise and Fall of Jim Crow: a PBS resource that includes videos and biographies of several of the scholars mentioned in this chapter (Ida B. Wells and W.E.B. DuBois) and details on the contributions of many others to challenge Jim Crow laws. http://www.pbs.org/wnet/jimcrow/stories_people.html

World Health Organization (WHO): an agency within the United Nations that monitors and addresses international public health. http://www.who.int/en/

References

Appelrouth, S. A., & Edles, L. D. (2012). *Classical and contemporary sociological theory* (2nd ed.). Los Angeles: SAGE.

Association of American Medical Colleges (AAMC). (2011). Preview guide for the MCAT 2015 exam. www.aamc.org/MCAT2015.

Association of American Medical Colleges (AAMC). (2012). Preview guide for the MCAT 2015 exam (2nd ed.). www.aamc.org/MCAT2015.

Berger, P., & Luckmann, T. (1966). *The social construction of reality*. New York: Doubleday.

Braveman, P., Egerter, S., & Williams, D. R. (2011). The social determinants of health: Coming of age. *Annual Review of Public Health, 32*, 381–398.

DuBois, W. E. B. (1903). *The souls of black folk*. New York: Penguin Books.

DuBois, W. E. B. (1920). *The souls of white folk*. New York: Prometheus Books.

Durkeim, E. (1897). *Suicide: A study in sociology*. New York: Free Press.

Frieden, T. R. (2013). CDC health disparities and inequalities report – United States, 2013. Centers for Disease Control and Prevention (CDC). *Morbidity and Mortality Weekly Report, 62*(3), 1–186.

Giddens, A., Duneier, M., Appelbaum, R. P., & Carr, D. (2014). *Introduction to sociology* (9th ed.). New York: W.W. Norton.

Healthy People. (2020). Social determinants of health. Available at: http://www.healthypeople.gov/2020/about/foundation-health-measures/Determinants-of-Health

Institute of Medicine (IOM). (2003). *Unequal treatment: Confronting racial and ethnic disparities in health care*. B. D. Smedley, A. Y. Stith, & A. R. Nelson (Eds.). Washington, DC: The National Academies Press.

Jones, P., Bradbury, L., & Le Boutillier, S. (2011). *Introducing social theory* (2nd ed.). Malden: Polity Press.

Marx, K., & Engels, F. ([1846] 1977). The communist manifesto. In R. C. Tucker (Ed.), *The Marx-Engels reader* (pp. 469–500). New York: W.W. Norton.

Mills, C. W. (1959). *The sociological imagination*. New York: Oxford University Press.

Morris, A. (2015). *The scholar denied: W.E.B. DuBois and the birth of modern sociology*. Oakland: University of California Press.

Weber, M. (1904). *The protestant ethic and the spirit of capitalism*. Translated by Talcott Parsons (1958). New York: Charles Scribner's Sons.

Chapter 2
Social Research Methods: Scientific Inquiry and Reasoning Skills in Social Science

Objectives

- Learn the major concepts and methodologies in social science
- Understand how scientific data is used and presented in social science research
- Evaluate research in social science critically
- Become a better informed user of the many social science studies that shape health policy

Foundational Concepts

"This section tests your knowledge and use of the concepts in psychology, sociology, biology, research methods, and statistics that provide a solid foundation for learning in medical school about the behavioral and socio-cultural determinants of health and health outcomes (AAMC 2015:8)".

The exam includes a section that tests your knowledge in the use of concepts including those related to research methods and statistics as they are applied in the social sciences. Understanding of how behavioral and socio-cultural determinants of health are formally studied in research is an essential skill to those who study medicine.

Included are Four Skills that Natural and Social Scientists Rely on to Advance Their Work. They Are:

Knowledge of Scientific Concepts and Principles
Scientific Reasoning and Problem Solving
Reasoning about the Design and Execution of Research
Data-Based and Statistical Reasoning

Source: *AAMC 2015*

G. Garcia-Alexander et al., *Social Foundations of Behavior for the Health Sciences*,
DOI 10.1007/978-3-319-64950-4_2

This chapter is designed to help you learn how to ask research questions and find answers, in a scientific and highly ethical way. In this chapter, we will cover important concepts and principles in research methods used in the social sciences. After introducing the key concepts, you will learn how to choose a method appropriate for a research question, conduct analysis to address the research question, and disseminate the findings. In each section, a number of examples on research areas and topics that are highly relevant to health research are provided.

2.1 Sociological Inquiry

Sociologists are always interested in learning about the social world. To do this, they formally develop and ask questions about the social world, and investigate them to find the answers. Can you think of any questions about the social world as an example? What about the use of the Internet? I am sure all of you have access to the Internet and today, it is almost impossible to do school work without it. Although course lectures may take place in a classroom, we heavily rely on the Internet for a number of course related activities. Professors make the course materials available on online course portals. Students no longer hand in their homework assignment to the professors. Rather, they turn in their work online. In addition, students communicate with professors via email or through the course website. These are just a small sampling of online activities that most, if not all of you engage in on a daily basis.

Accordingly, some questions about the Internet may arise and could be investigated in a sociological way. Examples include: (1) Do all American have access to the Internet?; (2) If not, which social group(s) are more likely to use the Internet compared to other social groups?; (3) Among those who have access to the Internet, are the levels of usage the same?; and (4) Is there any association between Internet use and individual health? (5) Does Internet use improve health or deteriorate it?

Can you answer these questions? You may have some thoughts or ideas about the correct answers. However, it is important to develop skills in finding the right sources of information, as well as how to both digest it and report it in a responsible way. To address the first and second questions, we might turn to existing statistics provided by a reputable survey center or organization. Some examples include places like the PEW Research Center, the Inter-university Consortium for Political and Social Research (ICPSR), the Census Bureau, and so on. As an example, in a recent report prepared by File, about 75% of U.S. households had a computer at home and almost as many had access to the Internet (File 2013). Internet use varies considerably by social groups as well. While 90% of those with at least bachelor's degree use the Internet, only 32% of those with less than a high school education use it (File 2013). Higher proportions of Internet use are also found among those with a higher household income and non-Hispanic whites and Asian Americans, compared to those with a lower family household income and Hispanics and non-Hispanic blacks (Cooper and Gallager 2004; Strickling 2010).

Answering the third and the fourth questions are not as straightforward as they may seem. The answers may depend on how we measure 'Internet use' and 'health,' and the modes of Internet use (i.e. smart phone, tablet, and pc). Thus, as social scientists, we would need to develop measures that represent our concepts, decide how we would obtain the data needed to answer the questions, and conduct some form of analysis to obtain a valid and reliable answer.

Social research methods are designed to reduce as much error and bias as possible in the way we ask and answer research questions. To consider this a bit further – are these answers surprising to you? Did you imagine different answers based on your personal experience? Do these variations make you cautious about using your own experience as a basis to answer these questions? Our social world is complex, and we cannot avoid asking questions to better understand our position in it. At the same time, our own experiences and opinions may influence the way we perceive and interpret the world around us. When our own experiences interfere with reasoning about the social world, this may lead to overgeneralization of the social world based on a limited (and often selective) exposure to the social world.

Sociological research methods allow us to investigate individuals, societies, and social processes in scientific ways while avoiding errors in reasoning about the social world. One type of error is when one relies too heavily on their individual observations, and applies those views to more than they are applicable. Thus, *overgeneralization* occurs when we assume that what is true for some is true for all. Another type of error results from making *selective* or *inaccurate* observations. For example, when people choose to look only at things that are in line with our preferences or beliefs, they have engaged in selective observation. We make errors of inaccuracy when we use *illogical reasoning*. This can happen when people jump to conclusions or base an argument on invalid assumptions. It may also occur if people use faulty logic to understand the patterns observed in the data. This is because the data itself is bias free – while our own thoughts and beliefs are not.

2.2 Key Concepts and Principles

Social research starts with inquiries about the social world that one (a researcher) would like to understand. The motivation or topic area may come from someone's firsthand experience. However, valid sociological research seeks to understand people within groups (rather than as an individual) and social processes (rather than an individual's unique experience). It can be useful to let your own experiences shape your research interests, but it should not influence your findings or outcomes. Social research is thus designed to remove as much possibility for bias to enter the research as possible. In order to specify a social research question, you need to: (1) identify a social problem or issue that influences a large group of people; (2) review existing relevant studies to learn what is already known about the social problem; and (3) following review of the literature, refine the research question to address what still needs to be answered.

Once the prior studies in the area have been reviewed, a theoretical framework should also be constructed. This helps to frame the argument and connect it to work that has already been done. In many instances, social researchers may attempt to support or refute theoretical arguments that might explain the presence of some social issue. Following this background development and framing, the researcher should proceed with the execution of the research.

In conducting research, sociologists strive to link empirical research findings to generalizable theory. Researchers make this link by starting with an existing social theory and testing a hypothesis (which is developed from the theory) with data. This approach is **deductive** in nature. This means we take a top-down approach by starting with some pre-existing theoretical assumptions and using those to make predictions about what the outcomes will be. Alternatively, researchers may first collect the data and then develop a theory based on findings from the data. We call this approach **inductive** reasoning.

In deductive research, researchers should have a specific expectation (i.e. hypothesis) based on the previous research, and test the hypothesis to learn about whether and how two or more variables are associated. In other words, a change in one variable (i.e. independent variable) is proposed to predict changes in the outcome variable (i.e. dependent variable). In contrast, inductive research starts with very general ideas about patterns and expectations. Then, the researcher allows the data (that often times the researcher collected) and observations to guide their understanding of how social concepts relate to one another. Thus in opposite fashion, they induce a general explanation from the data itself without applying pre-existing ideas or theories (Fig. 2.1).

In both strategies, the goal of social research is to improve our understanding about the social world by offering valid associations between social relations that may be applied to a large group of people or a society. Therefore, it is important to achieve **causal validity** (or **internal validity**), which refers to the idea that the approach used by the researcher produces results that are genuine and/or legitimate. **Generalizability** (or **external validity**) is the extent to which the outcomes generated may be used to inform us about people, public places, and social events/activities that were not studied or sampled. In other words, it refers to the idea that our results apply beyond the people or units that were studied in the sample.

Issues of validity and reliability are also important in the measurement of social phenomena. **Validity** in measurement refers to whether a variable measures exactly what it is intended to measure. This may be thought of as the accuracy of a measure in capturing what it is meant to. **Reliability** in measurement means that a measurement applied to the same object yields the same result each time. This may be thought of as the consistency of a measure in capturing a concept.

Validity and reliability in measurement go hand in hand, and both are needed to achieve solid research outcomes. When we measure the same thing repeatedly, but it is not necessarily an accurate measure of what we want to capture – we have achieved reliability but not validity. When we accurately capture a concept, but cannot consistently measure it in repeated tries – we have achieved validity but not reliability. Thus, we ultimately want our measures to be both consistent and accurate. These concepts are illustrated below (Fig. 2.2).

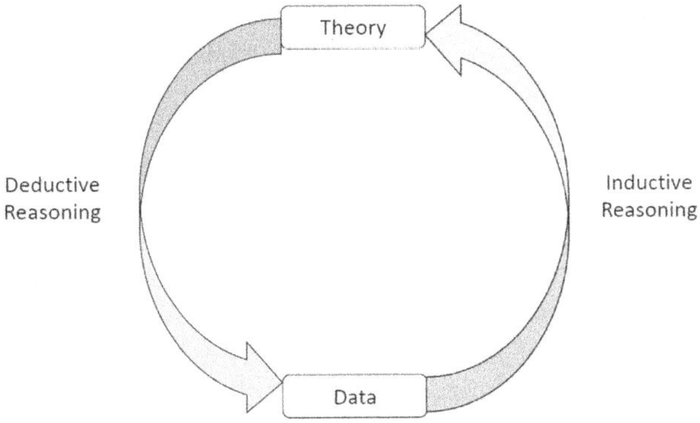

Fig. 2.1 Deductive and inductive reasoning

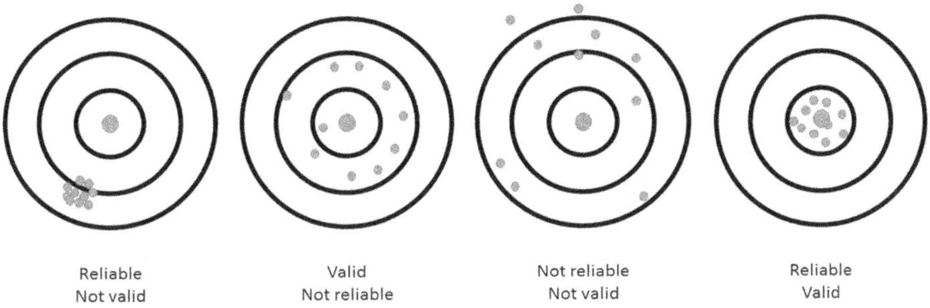

Fig. 2.2 Validity and reliability

2.2.1 How Do We Ensure Measurement Validity and Reliability?

Measurement validity can be broken down into three related concepts: (Face; Content; and Construct Validity. These three criterion are often used to ensure measurement validity. **Face validity** is achieved when a measure reflects the concept we want to capture "on its face" (Schutt 2015: p. 133). In other words, we can say that a measure is face valid if it clearly represents the concept, which is measured (Brewer and Hunter 1989). Weight and height are examples of face valid measures to study body mass index, as they represent an objective measure of the size of a human body. However, it should also be noted that face validity does not guarantee our research to be free of measurement error, as people may under-report their weight or over-report their height. **Content validity** exists when the full range of a concept's meaning is covered by the measure. For example, researchers often use a combination of the items related to emotional well-being from the Center for Epidemiologic Studies Depression Scale (CES-D) when measuring depression. As mentioned above, the CES-D items contain a range of questions related to this issue, ranging from mood-related questions to somatic symptoms to cover the full range depressive symptoms. Most social scientists will combine these items to create an index of depression that covers responses about a person's sleep patterns, their amount of hopeless thoughts, their level of isolation, and so on. Thus, the CES-D items have been widely used to measure depression in social science because they cover the full spectrum of symptomatology, thus achieving content validity. **Construct validity** refers to the degree to which a measure relates to other measures as expected or specified in a theory. This type of validity is useful to measure a concept that involves a lot of subjectivity, such as marital quality. The typical items used to measure marital quality include: (a) how much does your spouse make you feel loved and cared for? (b) how much is your spouse willing to listen to you?; (c) how often would you say you have disagreements or conflicts?; and (d) how often do you feel bothered or upset by your marriage? While neither face validity nor content validity approaches can be used for these items measuring marital quality, researchers observe that the items for support and conflicts are more strongly interconnected than other measures were. These connections occur in ways that would be expected based on existing theory, and thus provide indirect evidence that they are useful as a measure marital quality.

Measurement reliability also contains various sub-types including test-retest; alternate-forms; split-halves; and interobserver/intercoder. We can ensure measurement reliability (consistency of our measure) by testing the measure and then retesting it later to see if the results are the same or similar (i.e. **test-retest**). Or, researchers can also use slightly different versions of the questions (i.e. **alternate-forms**) to compare the results from the two versions of the questions. The researcher might do this by including two questions on a survey that are worded slightly differently, then comparing a person's answers to make sure they are consistent. Measurement reliability can be also established when researchers have the same (or similar) results after administering an instrument that has been separated into two parts to the same group of people (i.e. **split-halves**). Finally, when dealing with qualitative or non-numeric data, such as that obtained from interviews or focus groups, researchers must develop a way to maintain consistency in the way the responses are reviewed and interpreted. This is done to ensure that different members of the research team will code the data in the same way. Accordingly, consistency across different coders refers to **interobserver** or **intercoder** reliability. This helps to establish reliability while minimizing measurement error that may occur in data processing (i.e. **intero bserver/intercoder**).

2.2.2 *Concepts, Conceptualization, and Operationalization*

One of the most fundamental skills a social researcher must develop is the ability to identify and define their topic. A **concept** is a mental construct that represents some aspect of the world in simplified form with a set of similar observations, ideas, and feelings. Whether it is well defined or not, you can probably think of some examples for concepts. For example, what about depression? Can you define what depression means? To make these concepts useful in research, we have to define them through **conceptualization**, or the process of translating abstract ideas and images into specific variables that are measureable and testable in research. This definition can and should vary on the basis what the researcher intends. Thus, we must find an appropriate definition for our research purposes. For example, according to the Diagnostic and Statistical Manual of Mental Disorders (American Psychiatric Association 2013), depression is a mental illness that negatively affects how you feel, the way you think and how you act. Depression takes two forms: mood for negative feelings and malaise for bodily states. Using items that capture whether a person is feeling sad or having a depressed mood, or experiences of changes in appetite and troubling sleeping (or sleeping too much), are all ways we can capture depression based on the associated definition. This can be further specified to indicate whether a person has any evidence of symptoms and if it is mild or severe. This is all part of the conceptualization process.

Operationalization is a related term that deals with the process of setting up the measures of variables and constants once we have defined and conceptualized them. Thus, this is the more concrete way of capturing the concept we want to and can be thought of as the actual measurement process. For example, we may have a concept, depression that we plan to measure using survey questions on mood and physical outcomes. We might ask a person how often they experience feelings of hopelessness (never, rarely, sometimes, or often). We can then use the information they provide us to assess their level of depression. Formally, the information we collect is transferred into some sort of data management system with each answer given by each person representing his or her response, or score, on a variable. A **variable** is anything that varies, with more than one possible value. For example, self-identified race and ethnicity is a variable with several values, such as non-Hispanic white, non-Hispanic black, Hispanic, non-Hispanic Asian, and others. In fact, almost everything in the world is a variable. It is also helpful to distinguish between dependent and independent variables, which are used to set up hypotheses. A **dependent** variable is one that is the focus or outcome of the research. In comparison, an **independent** variable is the one that is expected to influence the outcome. As an example, let's say we want to examine how a person's gender is related to their level of depression. We might hypothesize that women will have higher levels of depression. In this example, gender is the independent variable and depression is the dependent variable.

A related concept that tells us about the type of variable we have is level of measurement. Levels of measurement refer to the mathematical precision with which the values of a variable can be expressed. There are four (i.e. Nominal; Ordinal; Interval; and Ratio) levels. The first and simplest level is a *nominal* measure. These are qualitative, such as gender and race variables. What that means is that the information they provide has no numeric meaning. For example, when we ask for a person's race they might tell us they are non-Hispanic white, non-Hispanic black, Hispanic, and so on. These response categories are not numerically bigger or smaller than one another, they are simply different. Compared to nominal ones, *ordinal* measures offer additional information about the rank order among the categories of

Table 2.1 Math operations by the levels of the measurement

	Levels of measurement			
Appropriate math operations	Nominal	Ordinal	Interval	Ratio
= (≠)	Yes	Yes	Yes	Yes
> (<)		Yes	Yes	Yes
+ (−)			Yes	Yes
× (/)				Yes

a variable. For example, social class is indicated by upper class, middle class and working class. These types of variables tell us about whether a person's response is above or below another, but they do not tell us exactly how much higher or lower. *Interval* measures refer to the ones that offer not only rank order information but also mathematical interpretation for the distance between the values. Temperature is a good example. In ratio measures, there is always an absolute zero that is meaningful. In social science, most "count" variables are ratio measures. For example, the amount of income you earned last year or the number of visits to the doctor's office in the past year are examples of ratio measures.

The table above describes the hierarchical properties of measurement levels and appropriate operations by the levels of the measurement (Table 2.1).

2.3 Sampling

In social science, it is almost impossible to study the entire population of interest, and thus researchers are required to use a subset of the larger target population (i.e. **sample**) that should look like the target population in small scale. The results obtained from a good sample, meaning one that was randomly selected and representative, can be generalized to the population from which the sample was selected. The individual members of this sample are called **elements** and to select these elements, we often rely on some list of all elements in the population, called *sampling frame*. How do we ensure that we have a good sample? There are several methodological approaches to consider.

Depending on whether the probability of selection of population elements is known, there are two different approaches for sampling: Probability sampling methods and non-probability sampling methods.

2.3.1 Sampling Methods: Probability Sampling

Probability sampling methods include four different types: simple random; systematic random; cluster; stratified random. Each of these methods is characterized by the use of randomly selected elements (random selection), which ensures that each element has an equal probability of being included in the sample. This allows us to apply the principles of probability and make generalizations about the population from which it was drawn with a certain level of confidence. Thus the larger the sample, the more confidence we can have in the sample's representativeness. Also, the more homogeneous the population, the more confidence we can have in the representativeness of a sample of any particular size. There are four sampling strategies for probability sampling methods. **Simple random sampling** is a method of sampling in which every sample element is selected on the basis of chance through a random process, like assigning a number to each person in the sampling frame and then using a random number generator to identify those who will be included in the sample. **Systematic random sampling** adopts a systematic way (e.g. selecting every *n*th element from a list or from sequential files) to randomly select the elements. In **cluster sampling**, elements are selected in two or more stages, with the first stage being the random selection of naturally occurring clusters (e.g. states) and the last stage being the random selection of elements within clusters (e.g. counties). In general, the more clusters you select, with the fewest individuals in each, the more representative your sampling will be. While it may provide a better coverage of the elements from various groups in the target population, sampling error tends to be greater in cluster sampling than in a simple random sampling. **Stratified random sampling** ensures researchers can represent various groups by using population strata that are identified in advance by the researcher. Demographic characteristics, such as gender, race/ethnicity, and age are often used to select elements either proportionately or disproportionately. For example, let's say the researcher was interested in focusing on Native Americans. Because this group is relatively smaller than other groups, the researcher might choose to oversample this group to be sure they have adequate responses. For disproportionate samples, weighting may be applied to make the sample representative to the target population.

2.3.2 Sampling Methods: Non-probability Sampling

Nonprobability sampling methods include availability, quota, purposive, and snowball. Nonprobability sampling methods are often used in qualitative research, or when researchers are unable to use probability selection methods. This sampling approach is useful for an intensive investigation of a small population or for a preliminary, exploratory study. There are four specific methodologies for nonprobability sampling methods. **Availability sampling** (or convenience sampling) refers to sampling in which elements are selected on the basis of convenience. In other words, the researcher chooses people they can easily get access to. **Quota sampling** is a nonprobability sampling method in which elements are selected to ensure that the sample represents certain characteristics in proportion to their prevalence in the population. Another strategy is **snowball sampling**, in which sample elements are selected as they are identified by successive informants or interviewees. Lastly,

purposive sampling can be used to select elements for a purpose, usually because of their unique position and knowledge about situation or experience being studied.

2.3.3 Causal Relationships

Sociologists like to observe various social issues and try to understand what may explain them. For example, disparities in longevity have been pressing public health concerns in the US, and educational differences across individuals have received much attention as one of the main reasons for this (Cutler and Lleras-Muney 2014; Kitagawa and Hauser 1973; Ross and Mirowsky 1999, 2003; Ross and Wu 1995). Based on this, is it safe to say education *causes* mortality? When deciding whether a causal relationship exists, three criterion must be considered: (1) Association; (2) A proper time order; and (3) Non-spuriousness. **Association** refers to a relationship where variation or a change in one variable (independent variable) is related to variation in another variable (dependent variable). When determining whether an association between two variables is causal, one must also occur before the other (i.e. **a proper time order**). Lastly, in order to establish a causal relationship, the association must not be spurious (i.e. **non-spuriousness**). Spuriousness refers to an association between two variables that is actually the result of a third variable.

Now let's go back to our research finding that those with higher levels of educational attainment tend to live longer – based on what we know about causality, can we say there is an association between education and mortality? If education is the independent variable and mortality is the dependent, we should also consider time order. It is clear that most of times individuals complete their education before an event of death (i.e. a proper time order). Finally, is the association between education and mortality caused by a third variable? In other words, is the relationship between education and mortality spurious or genuine? There are other conditions affecting education and mortality at the same time, such as parental education. That is, those whose parents have higher levels of education are more likely to have higher levels of education. Additionally, parents' higher levels of education also positively influence longevity of their children through more supportive parent-children relationship, better material support and healthier environment that they can provide for the children compared to parents with lower levels of education. However, the previous research confirms that parents' education is a precursor and the association between education and mortality is not spurious.

2.4 Research Design and Execution of Research

Now we turn to a review of several of the main research methods in social science – these represent the approaches social scientists use to empirically investigate hypotheses. We begin with experiments, then move on to qualitative methods, and end with a discussion of quantitative approaches.

2.4.1 *Experiments*

Experiments have always been a key method of scientific research, including social science. Key components of the experiment include clearly defined research question(s), independent and dependent variables, and successful experiments should control the conditions in which a hypothesis is tested and measure variables precisely (Willer and Walker 2007). In true experiments, study subjects are randomly assigned to an experimental group and a comparison group. Subjects in the experimental group receive a treatment or other manipulation of the independent variable, while subjects in the comparison group do not receive the treatment or other manipulation of the independent variable. After some exposures of the treatment (or other manipulation) among subjects in an experimental group, the researcher can compare the outcome of the dependent variable in a pretest and posttest from subjects of experimental and comparison groups.

Threats to Internal Validity (Causality). There are several points to ensure internal validity in experimental design. First, it is critical to have **comparable groups** for experimental and comparison groups. The groups should not have selection bias or differential attrition (dropping out of the study) during the study period. Also, a researcher should be aware of any external events (i.e. **history** during the experiment) that possibly influences the participants and the study outcomes, by making sure the different outcomes in post-tests between the experimental and comparison group is the result of the treatment, rather than the external event(s). Another issue is a possible endogenous change (i.e. **maturation**) in the experiment subjects, especially when the experiment involves a lengthy period. Over the treatment period, the subjects age, experience, and gain knowledge that may lead the subjects to alter their attitudes, opinions and responses for the posttest. When the subjects in the comparison group are in contact with the subjects in the experimental group (i.e. **contamination**) while the study is in progress, the subjects in one group may be affected by or affect the ones in the other group, and this contamination may also influence the posttest results. The subjects in the comparable group may believe that they have been left out of receiving some valuable treatment, and as a result, they may feel demoralized or make more efforts to compensate for this denial. Researchers should also be careful about potential threats that may occur in the form of a **self-fulfilling prophecy**, **placebo effects** and **Hawthorne effect**, which results in unexpected outcomes. In the case of self-fulfilling prophecy, this is when something happens because people expect it to. In the case of research, we have to be careful to avoid letting our expectations influence the outcome. This is often done in an experiment by using a double blind strategy so the researcher doesn't know who is in the treatment and who is in the control group. A placebo effect is when people who did not receive the treatment alter their own outcomes because they believe they are being treated. Finally, the Hawthorne effect is when people's behavior or outcomes change not because of the treatment or manipulation, but because they are aware they are being observed.

Threats to External Validity (Generalizability). It is more challenging to achieve external validity (i.e. generalizability) in experimental research given the artificial conditions of experiment. However, researchers should still attempt to increase generalizability by recruiting participants carefully to reflect the population of the study interest and assigning them randomly into the groups. Selecting several different experimental sites may also help. Even with well-recruited subjects and multiple study sites, researchers should also be aware of possible interaction effects between testing and treatment that occur among the subjects. During the pretest, the study subjects might become aware of the purpose of the study, and thus they might sensitize themselves in responding in the post-test.

Experimenting often serves as the primary tool for studying causal relationships and requires relatively little time and money. However, because it occurs in its artificial experimental lab setting (rather than a natural setting), the results are not necessarily readily applicable to the social world. Another drawback is that experimental research designs often involves more limitations from Institutional Review Board (IRB). More about the IRB is explained later in this chapter.

2.5 Qualitative Methods

Qualitative methods refer to several research approaches that are characterized by a higher level of detail and a focus on the quality of responses in relatively fewer participants. A group of anthropologists and sociologists laid the foundation for modern qualitative methods while doing fieldwork in the early twentieth century (Schutt 2015). These researchers went to the communities they studied and often lived there for a while to collect firsthand information about the natural behaviors of participants and artifacts that capture social life as participants experience it. Qualitative research designs share several features that distinguish them from other research designs, such as experimental and survey research designs.

- Qualitative approaches emphasize collecting qualitative data, capturing social behaviors as participants experience it – what people think, and how and why they act in social setting. In addition, qualitative data are not converted into categories that the researcher predetermines.
- Qualitative approaches are typically well suited for exploratory research questions, meaning those that have not been studied previously. Qualitative approaches

allow researchers to develop general principles to account for their observations once data is analyzed (i.e. inductive reasoning), rather than to test pre-formulated hypotheses (i.e. deductive approach).

- Qualitative designs tend to focus on human subjectivity, how study participants attach to events of research interests and how their lives are influenced.
- A research design and focus often takes an adaptive form as the research progresses.
- A researcher's subjectivity is sensitive to the research setting. Unlike quantitative methods, the role of the researcher may affect every aspect of the research – research design, creating rapport with participants, data quality, data analysis, and even findings of research.

The qualitative approach includes several different methods: participant observation, intensive interviewing, and focus groups. Each are described below.

2.5.1 Participant Observation

This method refers to a qualitative approach that collects data by observing individuals as they go about their normal activities. The researcher acts as a participant and as a member of the group.

Different Roles of a Qualitative Researcher. A researcher can adopt different roles while observing subjects. As a **covert observer**, a researcher observes study participants without participating in social events and activities, and does not self-identify as a researcher. This role may be adopted in public places where someone can sit and observe other people without appearing unusual or interfering with normal activities. However, in many cases, a qualitative researcher may function as a **complete observer**, who would observe activities without participating in them, but identify as a researcher. Unlike these passive roles, a qualitative research can be a complete participant (in other words, a covert participant) who participate in activities just like other study participants without disclosing the researcher's identity as a researcher. **Overt participants** (or, **participant observer**) refers to a qualitative researcher who identifies her/him as a researcher but nonetheless participates in social activities.

Procedures (Sampling/Data Collection). In participant observation, most researchers tend to limit their focus to just one or a few sites because they study the participants, places and the context of the events/activities intensively. Thus, sampling people and events/activities are based on several criteria, such as (1) whether people or sites can provide rich information pertaining to the research question; (2) whether people or sites can serve as a reference; and (3) whether people or sites provide a useful contrast (Kuzel 1999). There are several sampling strategies, including **availability sampling**, **quota sampling**, **purposive sampling** and **snowball sampling** (More detailed information about each sampling method was provided earlier in this chapter). Once the sample is created/recruited, **taking notes** is the primary means of collecting data from the participant observation (Emerson et al. 1995). Of course, it does not mean that the researchers should just take notes intensively while engaged in the field, as it would be disruptive. Rather, they should **jot down** main points and brief notes. Based on these notes, they typically write **comprehensive field notes** preferably within the next 24 h. Still pictures, videotapes, and printed materials circulated and posted can also serve as supplemented data sources.

2.5.2 Intensive Interviewing

Intensive (or in-depth) interviewing is another qualitative research method used to learn about people's experiences, thoughts and feelings. Researchers can do intensive interviewing during participant observation, but intensive interviewing can also be done by itself. Similar to participant observation, the main purpose of doing an intensive interview is to learn about people's experience of events/activities that interest researchers on the subject's own terms and in the contexts of their circumstances. Therefore, intensive interviewing and participant observation share several important common traits, such as developing and maintaining a **reciprocal relationship** with the interviewees. This type of relationship, in which both parties benefit, is critical in intensive interviewing and sampling strategies.

Questionnaires. Most (if not all) of us have likely taken a questionnaire (either short or long). Surveys usually contain two kinds of questions: multiple choice questions vs. open-ended questions. Unlike the more structured interviewing in a questionnaire, in intensive interviewing, researchers usually rely on **semi-structured questionnaires** with **open-ended questions**. During the interview, researchers usually have a few simple questions to gather background information while building **rapport**. Then a few general open-ended questions that are meant to derive more lengthy narratives are asked. By using open-ended questions, researchers take a more obtrusive role in developing a relationship with interviewees to have a comprehensive understanding of the interviewee's background, attitudes, experiences, and perceptions regarding the actions/events of interest from the interviewee's perspectives. Using a less structured questionnaire with open-ended questions, researchers have to be free to follow the data where they lead (Rubin and Rubin 1995) until the **saturation point** is reached. **Theoretical saturation** is the phase in which the researcher has continued sampling and analyzing until they can gain no new data, and the theory and concepts derived from the data are well-developed.

Data Collection. Researchers should have a few main questions and an outline of the interview topic for intensive interviews, and interviews can be a conversation between an interviewer and an interviewee. Tape recorders are commonly used to record intensive interviews. They allow the researcher to show adequate levels of interest and appreciation while ensuring less interrupting of the interviewee.

2.5.3 Focus Groups

Focus groups are groups of unrelated individuals that are formed by a researcher and then led into group discussion of a topic for 1 to 2 h (Krueger and Casey 2009). Using focus groups, a researcher asks specific questions and guides the discussion to ensure that the focus group participants provide information to address the questions. This approach is considered more cost effective as a means to gather in-depth information from several participants at once. However, because focus groups rely on group discussion to gather information from the participants, it may not be the best strategy to study sensitive issues, especially when confidentiality cannot be ensured.

Sampling Participants. To recruit focus group members, researchers often seek out volunteers who have some knowledge or information pertaining to the topic of the research. While focus group members do not have to represent the target population, researchers should ensure: (1) they create a focus group with 5–10 members who share some key demographic characteristics; and (2) they avoid having any forms of authority over other participants, including supervisors, teachers, or parents who may alter opinions of the group members or hinder candid answers to the questions.

Roles of the Moderator. In focus groups, several important roles are expected of the moderator. First, focus group moderators should start the discussion by introducing the importance of the topic and make clear that everyone in the focus group is expected to participate in the discussion. Second, it is important that moderators should take a neutral position that she/he does not favor any particular perspective or participant, so the members feel comfortable to express their opinions without having anyone dominating the discussion. Third, the moderator may start with simple and easy to answer general factual questions to generate interest in the topic, and then shift to key questions on specific issues. When discussing the issues, the moderator should handle any disagreement carefully so that participants continue discussing the issues without feeling unsafe or uncomfortable to participate.

2.5.4 Advantages and Limitations of Qualitative Research

Qualitative research is very advantageous to study populations that are hard to reach or are very limited in size. While focusing on a specific population or site, it allows researchers to comprehend the research participants and events/activities that the participants experienced with detailed information. On the other hand, qualitative research may not be generalized to a larger population. Often times, qualitative data is not replicable as it pertains to experiences and feelings of participants under specific social contexts. However, two ways of increasing generalizability in qualitative research are: (1) Choose the typical site(s) and study subjects that fit with typical situations, rather than choosing them out of researcher's convenience; and (2) Increase the number of interviewees and study sites, so some emerging patterns and findings can be validated (Schofield 2002).

2.6 Quantitative Methods

Quantitative research differs from qualitative in its emphasis on the use of deductive methods and generalizability. Quantitative researchers utilize large-scale samples and apply the principles of probability theory to generalize from their samples and make predictions about the larger population.

2.6.1 Surveys

The survey is a data collection method that utilizes a questionnaire. In survey research, a researcher can ask a wide range of questions that may be used for a number of research projects at relatively little cost. Also, surveys can be widely distributed to representative samples, which help in achieving generalizable results. Because of these reasons (versatility, efficiency, and generalizability), surveys are perhaps the most widely used method in sociological research. For a review of survey procedures refer to the booklet mentioned in the Resources section.

Modes of Survey Administration. There are various ways to administer the survey. A **mail-out survey** (self-administered surveys) is conducted by mailing a questionnaire to respondents who then administer the survey and mail it back to the researcher. While it is simple and cost efficient, the response rate is typically low. A **group-administered survey** is completed by individuals in a group setting. A response rate is not usually an issue for a group-administered survey. However, as it is conducted in a group setting, respondents may feel forced to participate in the survey or uncomfortable answering questions, especially if they are sensitive ones. In a **telephone survey**, researchers ask respondents questions over the phone and record the answers. Researchers obtain a sample from phone directories or commercial firms that provide files of the phone numbers. While it is still very popular, several concerns related to this method have arisen in recent years. People often are not home and it is difficult to get enough complete responses to make the results generalizable, even after multiple attempts of callbacks. Compared to the above methods, an **in-person interview** (using either 'paper and pencil' or 'computer assisted personal interviewing') is often considered the best survey design. Response rates are higher than with any other survey administration methods. Additionally, the questionnaire can be long and complex as clarifications from the interviewer can be provided as needed. Moreover, the survey administration environment and circumstances can be monitored. However, this method, as expected, costs more money and takes more time to complete compared to other methods. Lastly, an **electronic survey** (either through web surveys or email surveys) has become increasingly popular. Internet access has been widely available and many people use the Internet, making it possible to conduct large surveys, without geographic limitations. However, as Internet use is still more dominant among certain demographics (young, highly educated, middle-class, and professionals), a sampling for the general population can still be an issue (Tourangeau et al. 2012). A proper method should be selected depending on available funding and time, and the characteristics of a target population.

Advantages and Limitations of Survey Methods. In general, data collected using questionnaires is more easily quantified and analyzed than information generated by other research methods. As mentioned earlier, survey research is also advantageous when considering time and expense. However, compared to qualitative research, data gathered from survey research does not provide in-depth contextual information.

2.7 Quantitate Data Analysis

Statistics are essential to describe quantitative data collected from experimental or survey research, often expressed with certain mathematical concepts and techniques. This chapter gives a brief overview of the options for summarizing distributions, including measures of central tendency (mode; median; mean), and measures of variation (range; interquartile range; variance; standard deviation). These are referred to as descriptive statistics. Social scientists also use inferential statistics, which is the branch of statistics used to test whether results from a sample are generalizable to a larger population.

Measures of Central Tendency (i.e. mean, median and mode) are among the tools that social scientists use to describe the data they are analyzing. These measures are especially useful because they provide us with a single number that can be used to describe an entire group of people. The **mean** is an average, which is computed by dividing sum of the values of all the cases by the total number of cases. The **median** is the value in the middle in a distribution. The **mode** is the most frequent value in a distribution. It is used much less often than the other two measures of central tendency – mean and median, because it can easily provide misperception about central tendency when a distribution is bimodal.

Measures of Variation are another tool that can be used to tell us about how much variation, or difference there is between people's responses. Measures of central tendency provide incomplete summary of distributions, and without measures of variation, they can also be misleading. Measures of variation include, the **range**, or difference between highest value and lowest value. The **interquartile range** is computed by deducting the value of first quartile (the value corresponding to the first 25% of the cases) from the one of third quartile (the value corresponding to the first 75% of the cases). The **variance** is the average squared deviation of each case from the mean, and the **standard deviation** is the square root of the variance. Both variance and standard deviation account for the distance of each case from the mean.

The above measures are univariate, summarizing distributions of variables. Sociologists are also interested in associations between two or more variables, or whether or not things appear together more than would be expected by chance. To examine associations, **cross-tabulations**, **correlational analysis** and **multiple regression analysis** are commonly used. These types of measures allow us to consider more than one variable at a time and understand how they are related to one another.

2.8 Ethics in Research

Conducting research is a privilege, which allows you to better understand people and society, and through research, you contribute to a larger community in the hope of changing it for the better. While pursuing scientific knowledge is important, you should also be mindful of not only your research participants (including humans and non-humans), but also scientific disciplines, institutions, co-authors, fellow researchers, and people who read your research findings. Before we learn about how to protect them, you may wonder why we should protect humans and non-humans involved in research. Let us talk about this with a couple of examples that led to human suffering in the name of science.

In 1932, 600 African American men in Alabama joined the Tuskegee Syphilis Study by U.S. Public Health Service, believing that they were given free treatment. After funding for treatment was lost, the investigators continued the study until 1972 to follow the natural course of syphilis symptoms without treating the patients (see additional information on this issue in Chap. 6). More importantly, the patients were not informed that they were not treated. In fact, even when penicillin had become the standard treatment for syphilis by 1947, the scientists did not administer it to the patients. As you would imagine, the results were horrible – many of the men who participated in the study died, their wives contracted the diseases, and many of their children were born with congenital syphilis.

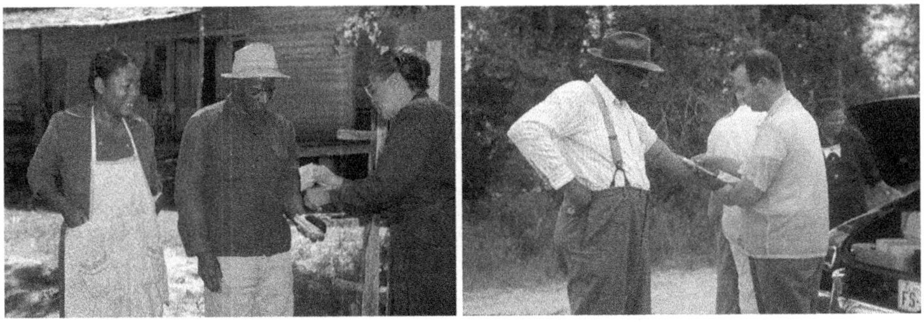

(Source: Centers for Disease Control and Prevention at https://www.cdc.gov/tuskegee/timeline.htm)

This is just one example of the harms committed under the heading of social research that led to the development of the following principles to protect human subjects: (1) protect research subjects; (2) to maintain honesty and openness; (3) achieve valid results; and (4) to encourage appropriate application (ASA 1997).

First, the most important ethical issue of protecting research subject may be achieved by: (1) avoiding anything that may potentially harm research participants; (2) obtaining informed consent from participants; (3) avoiding deception in research, except in limited circumstances where any ascertainable risk to subject is not expected; and (4) maintaining privacy and confidentiality after a study is completed. As for the second guideline to maintain honesty and openness, researchers have an obligation to do so by presenting and disseminating their findings, and by clearly describing their methods and findings. This is necessary to assess the validity of findings of a study. Ethical issues also apply to achieving valid results. Researchers should focus on pursuing objective knowledge by following scientifically justified procedures to produce knowledge; setting aside his/her own prejudices or pursuing their own personal interests.

Lastly, researchers should consider how their findings might be used/interpreted. Researchers may believe that once their findings are disseminated to the public, there is little to no concern about the way their research findings are used. However, as frequent use of one or more of social networking services has become more common in recent years, many people share research findings through various websites of social networking services, making it easy to misinterpret research findings, or use them in misleading ways. It is impossible for researchers to fully control how their research findings should be interpreted, however, it is their ethical obligation to encourage the application of their findings appropriately and try to correct it when they are misinterpreted.

2.8.1 The Institutional Review Board

In order to review the ethical issues in all proposed research that is federally funded, involves human subjects, or has any potential for harm to human subjects, federal regulations require that every institution have an institutional review board (IRB). IRBs at universities and other agencies apply ethical standards that are set by federal regulations but can be expanded or specified by the institution's IRB and involve all research at the institution regardless of the funding source (Sieber 1992). The main role of the IRB is to determine whether a proposed study involves human subjects and whether it considers human subjects protections sufficiently.

Activities and Discussion Questions

- **Activity 1: Conducting Research in a Health Setting**
  Medical doctors have long been engaged in producing research. They often have hands on experience in rare cases of diseases/symptoms. Additionally, they often have access to patient data with detailed medical information through the hospital records. Form a group with two or three people including yourself for the following activities and discussion question.
  Suppose that you have a new drug for cancer treatment that needs to be tested. Can you design an experimental study? Specify clearly how the independent variable will be examined and how the dependent variable will be measured, and formulate recruitment for study subjects and procedures for group assignments. Also, think about ways to avoid (or minimize) threats of internal validity.
- **Activity 2: Sampling**
  Suppose that you have hospital records with about a million patient cases from which you can select a sample of 1000 cases. What sampling method(s) would you use to select your sample? How can you ensure reliability in your study sample?
- **Activity 3: Qualitative and Quantitative Research**
  Think of research topics for intensive interview and survey in health research, and provide justifications for why intensive interview and survey are appropriate approaches for the topics you think of. For each research method, what are the factors that need to be considered in executing it appropriately?
- **Discussion Question 1:** What are the potential challenges in complying with ethical guidelines in medical research?

Study Questions

1. **What are the main methods used by social scientists to study group behavior and social processes?**
2. **How do researchers define and measure their concepts? What is a variable?**
3. **How do social scientists identify samples?**

***Example Exam Question:** "Given the design of a study described in the passage, which independent variable is manipulated?

A. Participants' actual vulnerability to cancer.
B. Participants' perceived vulnerability to cancer.
C. Exposure to tan versus pale models.
D. Tanning history.

A subgroup of children in the control group completed the same tasks 2 weeks after their initial testing session. Comparing their performance to that at the initial testing session would provide evidence of the tasks:

A. Reliability
B. Reportability
C. Standardization
D. Validity" (AAMC 2012: 117)

*For more information, visit https://students-residents.aamc.org/applying-medical-school/article/whats-mcat-exam/

Resources and Links

ICPSR: ICPSR advances and expands social and behavioral research, acting as a global leader in data stewardship and providing rich data resources and responsive educational opportunities for present and future generations. It maintains a data archive of more than 250,000 files of research in the social and behavioral sciences. It hosts 21 specialized collections of data in education, aging, criminal justice, substance abuse, terrorism, and other fields. https://www.icpsr.umich.edu/icpsrweb/index.jsp

Roper Center for Public Opinion: The Roper Center for Public Opinion Research is one of the world's leading archives of social science data, specializing in data from surveys of public opinion. http://www.ropercenter.uconn.edu/

- iPoll: most comprehensive and up-to-date resource for US public opinion poll data; provides access to poll questions and direct links to datasets and questionnaires

Quick Health Data Online: Provides state and county data for all 50 states, the District of Columbia, and U.S. territories and possessions. Data sets are available by gender, race, and ethnicity that come from a variety of national and state sources. Includes demographics, mortality, natality, reproductive health, violence, prevention, disease, and mental health statistics. http://www.healthstatus2020.com/owh/

Key Terms

- **Deductive Research**: a reasoning approach starting with some pre-existing theoretical assumptions and use those to make predictions about what our outcomes will be
- **Inductive Research**: a reasoning approach starting with collecting data and then develop a theory based on findings from the data
- **Causal Validity (Internal Validity)**: the extent to which a particular technique applied to the project produces results that are genuine and/or legitimate
- **Generalizability (External Validity)**: the extent to which outcomes generated in a study can be used to inform about people, public places, and social events/activities that were not studied or sampled
- **Reliability**: reliability in measurement means that a measurement applied to the same object yield the same results each time
- **Validity**: validity in measurement refers to whether a variable measures exactly what it is intended to measure. The following three criterion are used to ensure measurement validity:
  - **Face Validity**: the extent to which a measure represents the concept clearly
  - **Content Validity**: the extent to which the full range of a concept's meaning is covered by the measure
  - **Construct Validity**: the extent to which the degree to which a measure relates to other measures as expected or specified in a theory
- **Variable**: anything that varies, with more than one possible value
- **Levels of Measurement**: the mathematical precision with which the values of a variable can be expressed
  - **Nominal**: qualitative measures without any numeric meaning
  - **Ordinal**: measures with responses that can be rank ordered
  - **Interval**: measures offering not only rank order information but also mathematical interpretation for the distance between the values
  - **Ratio**: most count measures are ratio where an absolute zero as a value is meaningful
- **Sample**: a subset of the larger target population that should look like the target population in small scale
- **Probability Sampling**: sampling methods that reply on a random selection method so that the probability of selection of population elements is known
  - **Simple Random Sampling**: Sampling method in which every sample element is selected only on the basis of chance through a random process

  - **Systematic Random Sampling**: Sampling method in which sample elements are selected from a list or from sequential files, with every *n*th element being selected after the first element is selected randomly within the first interval
  - **Cluster Sampling**: Sampling method in which elements are selected in two or more stages, with first stage being the random selection of naturally occurring clusters and the last stage being the random selection of elements within clusters
  - **Stratified Random Sampling**: Sampling method in which sample elements are selected separately from population strata that are identified in advance by the researcher

- **Non-Probability Sampling**: Sampling methods in which the probability of selection of population elements is unknown
  - **Availability Sampling (Convenience Sampling)**: Sampling method in which elements are selected on the basis of convenience
  - **Quota Sampling**: Sampling method in which elements are selected to ensure that the sample represents certain characteristics in proportion to their prevalence in the population
  - **Snowball Sampling**: Sampling method in which sample elements are selected as they are identified by successive informants or interviewees
  - **Purposive Sampling**: Sampling method in which elements are selected for a purpose, usually because of their unique position

- **Criterion for Causal Relationship**: When deciding whether a causal relationship exists, three criterion (i.e. association; a proper time order; and non-spuriousness) must be considered
- **Experiment**: Research design controlling the conditions in which a hypothesis is tested and measure variables precisely
- **Experimental Group vs. Comparison Group**: In experiments, study subjects in the experimental group receive a treatment or other manipulation of the independent variable, while study subjects in the comparison group do not receive the treatment or other manipulation of the independent variable
- **Participant Observation**: Qualitative method that collects data by observing individuals
- **Intensive Interviewing**: Qualitative method that collects data through in-depth interviewing
- **Focus Group**: Qualitative method that collects data from group discussion of the study participants
- **Surveys**: Quantitative method that collects data using a questionnaire
- **Mean**: average, which is computed by dividing sum of the values of all the cases by the total number of cases
- **Median**: the value in the middle in a distribution
- **Mode**: the most frequent value in a distribution
- **Range**: a difference between highest value and lowest value
- **Variance**: the average squared deviation of each case from the mean
- **Standard Deviation**: the square root of the variance

- **Institutional Review Board (IRB)**: institutional committee that reviews the ethical issues in all proposed research that is federally funded, involves human subjects, or has any potential for harm to human subjects.

References

American Psychiatric Association. (2013). *Diagnostic and statistical manual of mental disorders* (5th ed.). Arlington: American Psychiatric Association.

Association of American Medical Colleges (AAMC). (2012). *Preview fuide for the MCAT 2015 exam* (2nd ed.). www.aamc.org/MCAT2015.

ASA. (1997). *Code of Ethics at the ASA* website www.asanet.org/about/ethics.cfm

Brewster, J., & Hunter, A. (1989). *Multimethod research: A synthesis of styles*. Newbury Park: Sage.

Cooper, K. B., & Gallagher, M. D. (2004). *A Nation Online: Entering the Broadband Age*. Washington, DC: Economics and Statistics Administration and National Telecommunications and Information Administration, U.S. Department of Commerce. Retrieved from the website at https://www.ntia.doc.gov/files/ntia/editor_uploads/NationOnlineBroadband04_files/NationOnlineBroadband04.pdf

Cutler, D., & Lleras-Muney, A. (2014). Education and health. In A. J. Culyer (Ed.), *Encyclopedia of health economics* (pp. 232–245). Cambridge, MA: Elsevier.

Emerson, R. M., Fretz, R. I., & Shaw, L. L. (1995). *Writing ethnographic Fieldnotes*. Chicago: University of Chicago Press.

File, T. (2013). Computer and internet use in the United States. In *Current population survey reports* (pp. 20–569). Washington, DC: U.S. Census Bureau.

Kitagawa, E. M., & Hauser, P. M. (1973). *Differential mortality in the United States: A study in socioeconomic epidemiology*. Cambridge, MA: Harvard University Press.

Krueger, R. A., & Casey, M. A. (2009). *Focus groups: A practical guide for applied research* (4th ed.). Thousand Oaks: Sage.

Kuzel, A. J. (1999). Sampling in qualitative inquiry. In B. F. Crabtree & W. L. Miller (Eds.), *Doing qualitative research* (2nd ed., pp. 33–45). Thousand Oaks: Sage.

Mirowsky, J., & Ross, C. E. (1999). Economic hardship across the life course. *American Sociological Review, 64*, 548–569.

Mirowsky, J., & Ross, C. E. (2003). *Education, social status and health*. Hawthorne: Aldine De Gruyter.

Ross, C. E., & Chia-ling, W. (1995). The links between education and health. *American Sociological Review, 60*, 719–745.

Rubin, H. J., & Rubin, I. S. (1995). *Qualitative interviewing: The art of hearing data*. Thousand Oaks: Sage.

Schofield, J. W. (2002). Increasing the Generalizability of qualitative research. In A. Michael Huberman & M. B. Miles (Eds.), *The qualitative Researcher's companion* (pp. 171–203). Thousand Oaks: Sage.

Schutt, R. K. (2015). *Investigating the social world*. Thousand Oaks: Sage.

Sieber, J. E. (1992). *Planning ethnically responsible research: A guide for students and internal review boards*. Thousand Oaks: Sage.

Strickling, L. E. (2010). *Digital National: 21st Century America's Progress Toward Universal Broadband Internet Access. An NTIA Research Preview*. Washington, DC: National Telecommunications and Information Administration, U.S. Department of Commerce. Retrieved from the website at https://www.ntia.doc.gov/files/ntia/publications/ntia_internet_use_report_february_2011.pdf

Tourangeau, R., Conrad, F. G., & Couper, M. P. (2012). *The science of web surveys*. Oxford: Oxford University Press.

Willer, D., & Walker, H. A. (2007). *Building experiments: Testing social theory*. Stanford: Stanford University Press.

Chapter 3
Self-Concept and Identity Development

Objectives

- Introduce sociological perspectives on the development of self-identify and its stages
- Discuss the role of social processes in identity formation and self-presentation
- Understand how self-concept and identity influence human behavior

Foundational Concept 8
Psychological, sociocultural, and biological factors influence the way we think about ourselves and others.

Category 8C (*social processes*) how the presence of others focuses on attitudes and beliefs that affect social interactions including prejudice, bias, and stereotyping.

"Social thinking refers to the ways in which we view others and our environment, as well as how we interpret others' behaviors. A variety of factors – personality, environment, and culture – factor into the beliefs and attitudes we develop" (AAMC 2012: 107).

Category 10A (*social interactions*) focuses on the actions and processes underlying social interactions and discrimination.

"Human beings are social by nature. Though the sentiment is simple, the actions and processes underlying and shaping our social interactions are not" (AAMC 2012: 108).

People are sensitive to how they are seen by others while interacting in a social setting. Individuals develop their identities – who they are and what is meaningful to them – through the life course. In Sociology, two types of identity are considered: **social identity** and **self-identity**. In this chapter, we define both social identity and

G. Garcia-Alexander et al., *Social Foundations of Behavior for the Health Sciences*, DOI 10.1007/978-3-319-64950-4_3 self-identity, outline the development of identities, and review existing theoretical perspectives on the ways individuals view themselves and others. This information is vital to those in the health field given that it is needed to understand interactions and exchanges with both patients and colleagues. It also provides an understanding of how identity development varies and leads to differences that would potentially influence patient-provider interactions.

3.1 Self-Identity

Self-identity refers to the ongoing process of self-development through interactions between ourselves and the world around us over the life course (Giddens et al. 2016). People self-identify by various factors, including gender and race/ethnicity. These identities shape our interactions with others, how people view us, and our level of access to various resources.

Gender is a critical aspect of self-identity. While sex typically refers to males and females based on biological differences, gender refers to socially influenced differences between the sexes. Gender influences individuals' self-concept through the names they were given and how differently they are treated by parents as well as other people around them based on their gender (Leaper 2002). Several theoretical approaches have been introduced to the development of gender identity. For example, Sigmund Freud argued that infants and young children learn gender differences (i.e. masculinity and femininity) based on possession (or absence) of a penis. Boys form a rivalry relationship for the affections of their mother with father because they both possess a penis. On the other hand, girls relate with their mothers (who do not have penis) thus leading them to take on a submissive attitude. While this is considered an influential theory of the gender identity, a number of critiques have been raised against Freud's theory. The main critiques are that: (1) his view on gender difference is narrowly tied to whether one has penis or not; and (2) he makes the assumption that the penis is superior to the vagina with no real basis. Unlike Freud, Nancy Chodorow claimed that learning to be a male or female is derived from an infant's attachment to parents (especially the mother) during childhood. Girls stay close to their mother and develop their identity as a woman by relating to the mother. However, boys develop their identity by seeing themselves as different from their mother and then understanding masculinity as that which is not feminine. Like Freud, her theory is also criticized; mainly because it is based on a two-parent family structure whereby the mother is assumed to take care of children and the father is a sole breadwinner.

The above-mentioned gender development processes are based on gendered roles (often assumed to be naturally formed) observed during the early childhood. In contrast, West and Zimmerman (1987) view gender identity as resultant from what one does by "doing gender" in almost every social interaction – rather than what one is inherently (also see Chap. 4). Through interactions, individuals do and assess gendered behaviors, which maintain and reinforce the gender structure.

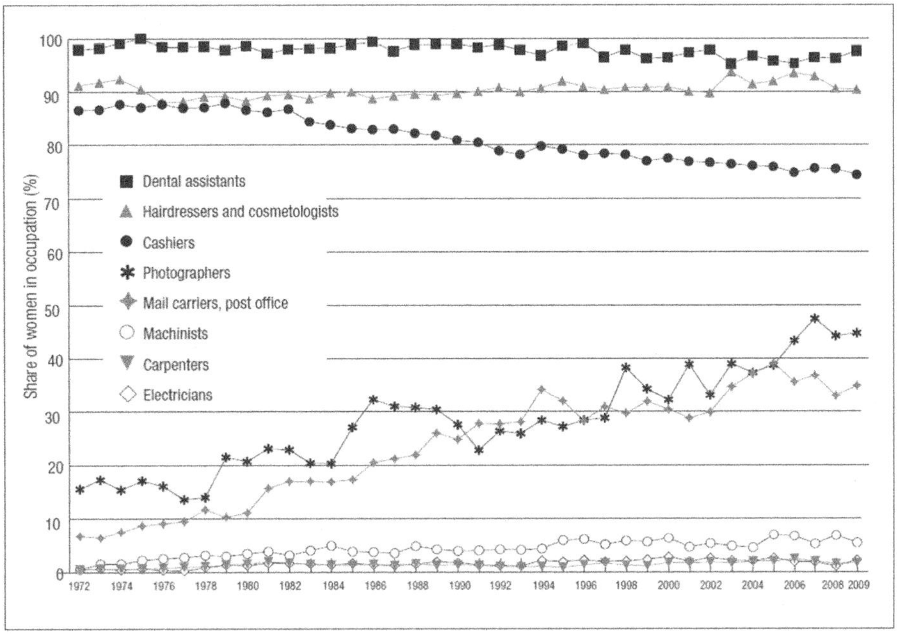

Notes: Data refer to annual averages and to all employed persons 16 years and older. From 2003 on, the category of 'hairdressers and cosmetologists' includes 'hair stylists' explicitly.

Source: IWPR compilation of data from the U.S. Department of Labor, Bureau of Labor Statistics, "B-20. Employed persons by detailed occupation, sex, and race, 1972-81;" "Employed persons by detailed occupation, sex, and race (1982);" "Employed persons by detailed occupation and sex, 1983-2002 annual averages;" "Employed persons by detailed occupation and sex, annual averages 2000-09." Data are from the Current Population Survey.

Fig. 3.1 Share of women in selected occupations requiring less than 4 years of college, 1972–2009 (Source: Hegewisch et al. 2010: p. 3)

Similarly, the *social cognitive perspective* also views gender identity development as a multifaceted process through interactions between personal and social factors, varying across individuals and across the life span (Bussey 2011). Unlike the previous theories, the social cognitive perspective sees the process as fluid rather than fixed, meaning people can develop their competencies and self-belief that are not mandated by their gender. As a result, gender roles continue to change. For example, increasing female presence in traditionally male dominant and more prestigious occupations has been observed in recent years. Figure 3.1 shows that while women are more likely to be in some occupations such as 'dental assistants' and 'hairdressers and cosmetologists,' the shares of women in such occupations as 'photographers' and 'mail carriers' have been increasing.

Similarly, in occupations that require at least a 4-year degree, there has been a blurring of gender segregation. As shown in Fig. 3.2 below, the proportions of women in some prestigious occupations, including pharmacists, physicians, surgeons, dentists, and lawyers, have been increasing. However, women are still dominant in occupations including teachers, registered nurses, and librarians. As gender roles become less distinctive and the genders are treated more equally, we may see that gender identity plays a less pervasive role in individuals' lives.

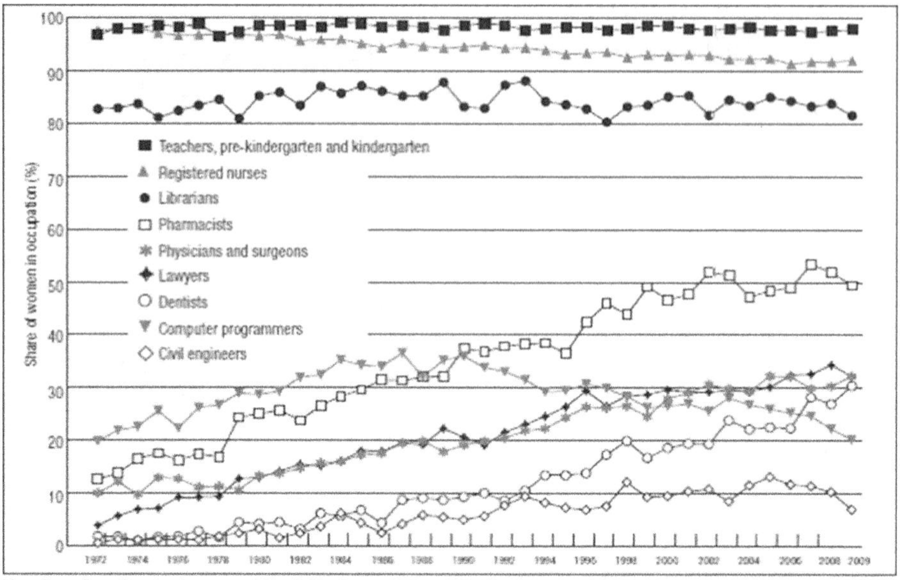

Notes: Data refer to all employed persons aged 16 and older. Between 1975 and 1982, 'physicians and surgeons' were described as 'physicians, medical and osteopathic' and between 1983 and 2002 as 'physicians.' The most common level of education for preschool teachers is a postsecondary vocational award while it is a Bachelor's degree for kindergarten teachers. After 2003, 'teachers, prekindergarten and kindergarten' were accounted for as 'preschool and kindergarten teachers.'

Source: IWPR compilation based on same data sources as Figure 1.

Fig. 3.2 Share of women in selected occupations requiring 4 years of college or more, 1972–2009 (Source: Hegewisch et al. 2010: p. 4)

Historically, gender identity was often viewed dichotomously, as one's sense of being male or female, based on biological sex. However, it is important to recognize other genders (e.g. **transgender**, or gender neutral). When one's gender identity and biological sex are not congruent, the individual may identity themselves as transgender or gender neutral (Gainor 2000). Alternatively, **cisgender** is used to refer to 'nontransgender,' – those whose biological sex and gender identity match (Schilt and Westbrook 2009). According to a recent report, approximately 0.6% of adults in the United States identify as transgender (Flores et al. 2016), but thanks to several public figures, such as Caitlyn Jenner, Laverne Cox, and Lana and Lily Wachowski (directors, formerly called "Wachowski brothers") just to name a few, the term of transgender has gained much awareness and greater acceptance. However, transgender individuals still face many challenges that are not experienced by cisgender people. One example, among others, is their right to access to public facilities. The Public Facilities Privacy & Security Act (commonly called "bathroom bill") has been signed in North Carolina in 2016, affecting access to public restrooms for the transgender people, and Texas also approved a similar measure.

3.1.1 *Racial/Ethnic Identity*

Social psychological theories emphasize how the social meanings members of society assign to racial and ethnic groups influence individuals in terms of attitudes and behaviors toward both those within the same racial and ethnic group and those outside the group. As Giddens et al. (2016) state, the social psychological approach is interested in looking at how individuals' perceptions of different groups affect their subsequent interactions with others, and how such interactions on the micro-level reflect and reshape relationships among racial groups at the macro-level.

While more detailed discussion on race and ethnicity is covered in Chap. 6, it is important to review how racial and ethnic prejudice present in society may affect individuals' behaviors and development of self. Prejudice is defined preconceived feelings (either positive or negative) toward people or a person because of their traits, such as race/ethnicity, gender, age, or other sociodemographic characteristic (Dovidio and Gaertner 2010). Prejudice often operates through stereotyping, referring to the adoption of simplified beliefs about specific types of individuals or certain ways of doing things, that are not necessarily based on scientific evidence (McGarty et al. 2002).

With respect to race and ethnicity, research has shown how prejudice against black students may lead them to underperform in school in two main ways. First, according to a study by Fordham and Ogbu (1986), the prejudice that white Americans hold against black students – which is often characterized by the belief that black students are not capable of intellectual achievements – creates **stereotypes**, which leads black students not only to doubt themselves but also to define academic success as that which is accepted by members of the dominant group in society. In turn, black students may experience or internalize these beliefs which lead to underperformance. This has also been shown to be the case in studies of academic *priming*. In these studies, researchers have shown that students who are *primed* with words suggesting they are highly intelligent actually do go on to outperform those who have not been *primed*. The second mechanism that can impact identity, subsequent perceptions, and interactions is **stereotype threat**, which is defined as a situational predicament where people feel at risk of conforming to existing stereotypes against the social group of which they are members. Stereotype threat occurs when people are aware of negative stereotypes about the social group of which they are a member, and experience anxiety that they may confirm and reinforce the stereotype. Steele and Aronson did an experiment to test the stereotype threat (Steele and Aronson 1995). In this experiment, they had college students take a verbal test. Importantly, when the test was introduced as an intelligence test, black students performed worse than their white counterparts did. However, when the test was not framed as an intelligence test, the gap between the black students and the white students reduced.

A recent report by Pew Research Center reveals that a substantial proportion of adults in the US have racial bias that exists at the subconscious level. This study examines the extent to which single-race individuals have a subconscious preference for the five racial groups, including both single-race (i.e. white, black and Asian) and biracial groups (i.e. white-black biracial and white-Asian biracial) (Fig. 3.3).

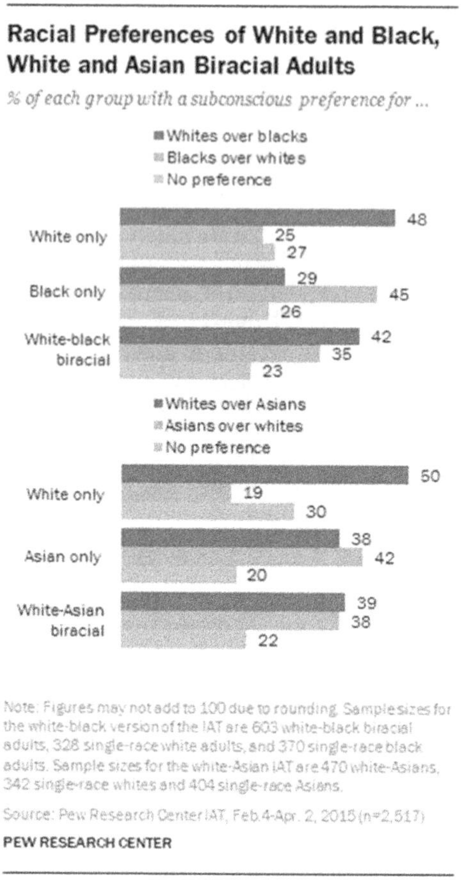

Fig. 3.3 Racial preferences (Source: Morin 2015)

According to the above figure, only about 20% to 30% of those in the study have little preferences toward the races they were tested against. For example, for single-race whites, almost a half of them prefer their own racial group (i.e. whites) over blacks (i.e. 48%) and only 25% prefer blacks over whites. Single-race blacks seem less biased compared to whites, but still a substantial proportion of them (i.e. 45%) prefer their own group over whites. Among white-black biracial group, 42% prefer whites over black, and 35% prefer blacks over whites. The racial bias toward Asian seems greater. Among whites, 50% prefer whites over Asians, and only 19% prefer Asians. Among Asians, while the difference between 'whites over Asians' and 'Asians over whites' is smaller, 80% indicated preference toward either whites or Asians. This pattern is similar to white-Asian biracial although a slightly higher proportion of them indicated preference to whites over Asians.

In addition to these theories for gendered processes of identity and racial/ethnic stereotypes affecting self-identities, it is important to recognize that the development and formation of self-identity are also influenced by various other factors, including academic performance, socioeconomic position, social relationships and networks, and sexual orientation through a lifelong complex process of socialization (See Chap. 4 for more information about socialization).

3.2 Life Stages

In most advanced contemporary societies, the overall life expectancy has been prolonged and thus, even after childhood, individuals experience a continuous development over the life course (Featherman 1983). According to the life course perspective, adults are also expected to develop multiple identities as they take on new social roles, and their social behaviors are also subject to be influenced through interactions with social agents in various social domains.

Based on major life transitions that are expected over the life span, the life stages to develop these identities are often divided into: *childhood*; the *teenager*; *young adulthood*; *mature adulthood*; and *old age*. **Childhood** refers to the life stage from infancy to the teen years. Childhood is critical to identity development as human beings undergo both physical growth and cognitive development. In this stage, human beings are exposed to a much larger social world outside of the family, and are engaged in extended social interactions with friends, peers, and teachers. Also, children start schooling to learn knowledge and skills necessary to be a member of the society. Over the **teenager stage**, people complete their physical growth while still receiving a formal education, and expanding their peer relationships and social realms. During **young adulthood**, several significant transitions into adulthood are expected to occur, including completion of education, getting a full time job, entry into marriage, and becoming a parent, which entailing multiple social roles. **Mature adulthood** is often characterized by changes in career, promotions at work, experiences of marital dissolution/remarriage and empty nest syndrome, and loss of parent(s). In mature adulthood, people may also start experiencing declines in health and physical functioning. During **old age**, people are expected to retire from work. Also, they may experience more health issues, declines of cognitive functioning, and bereavement of the spouse while their material resources and social networks may be reduced in size.

As would be expected, individuals consistently face changes in social roles that they are engaged with as the life stages unfold. The number of social roles expected to be taken changes as the responsibilities of the roles to be performed also are shifted. Social roles are linked to social identities, affect self-identities, and consequently shape and alter social behaviors.

3.2.1 Social Identity

Social identity refers to the characteristics that other people attribute to an individual, in accordance with various social roles; placing the individual with respect to others who share the same attributes (Giddens et al. 2016). All individuals have multiple social identities reflecting different roles at various dimensions of their lives. For example, someone could be a professor for her occupation, a researcher for various kinds of projects she conducts, a wife to her husband at home, and a mother to her child; and these social identities mark ways in which people are the same as others.

The following figure shows four statuses of one person that define identities, which are linked to different roles in various settings (Fig. 3.4). As you can see from the below figure, first, this woman is identified as a professor performing two roles: teaching students and interacting with colleagues for administration work for the department, university and other professional organizations that she is affiliated with. The second identity she has is a researcher. As a researcher, she collects and analyzes data (from her fieldwork) and writes about the findings (performing an author role). She also has a wife identity and a mother identity. As a wife, she shares domestic role to maintain the household with her husband and performs her marital role as a supportive confidante and a sexual partner toward her husband. Lastly, she raises her children (i.e. maternal role) and participates in parent's activities at her

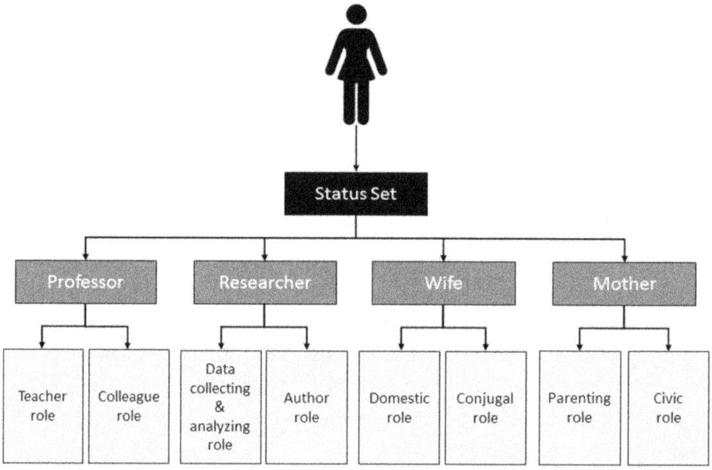

Fig. 3.4 Social statuses and roles

children's school (i.e. civic role). In performing multiple roles (e.g. as professor/researcher and wife/mother) in different settings (e.g. work and family domains), people often experience **role conflict** (conflict among the roles from two or more social identities) and **role strain** (strain among the roles connected to one social identity). People are constantly expected to adjust their social behaviors to perform roles in accordance with one role versus another.

Both self and social identities shape our interactions with others, how people view us, and our level of access to various resources. Below, we discuss how sociologists view an individual's social behaviors.

3.3 Self-Presentation

Sociologist Erving Goffman and others focus on the process by which people act and react to the people around them. For example, Goffman uses a theatrical setting to analyze human behaviors (i.e. **dramaturgical approach**). According to Goffman, people use many forms of **impression management**, preparation for the presentation of one's social role on a stage. Each social role brings different expected behaviors of people occupying particular social positions. In every society, individuals play a number of social roles.

3.3.1 Adopting Roles

Collaboration is a key component in impression management. Think of a situation involving a woman's visit to a male gynecologist's office. In the US, people are socialized that the genitals are the most private part of the body, and seeing and touching another person's genitals is usually associated with intimate sexual encounters. However, a series of behaviors typically occurring in the doctor's office suggest that people adopt a dramaturgical metaphor, in which the parts the actors play alter as the episode unfolds (Giddens et al. 2016: 94). For example, in the prologue, the woman enters the waiting room preparing to assume the role of patient. The next scene is at the consulting room where she adopts the "patient" role and the doctor assumes a role of medical professional. As the doctor leaves, the nurse comes in to help alter the patient from a person to a nonperson, so the private body part to be examined is an object to be scrutinized, free of sexual overtones. After the examination is over, the patient gets ready to wrap up the scene. The doctor may re-enter to discuss results of the examination, treating the patient in a polite and professional manner in an effort to assure her that his behaviors are not altered by the intimate contact with her private body part. As the patient leaves the doctor's office, she is ready to resume her identity in the outside world.

3.3.2 Theories of Social Interaction

Goffman argued that the study of **social interaction** offers important insights for human social life for three reasons. First, every day, routine interactions essentially serve as a foundation of what we do as social beings. Additionally, social interaction reveals the mechanisms of how human beings create/maintain reality. Social behaviors are guided by social norms and social role expectations shared by members of the society. However, individuals also have agency to think and act independently. These creative actions (re)shape reality through interactions with others. Lastly, studying individuals' behavior helps us understand larger societies.

A related concept is that of **personal space**, a concept expanded on by Edward Hall. Hall's main interest was in nonverbal communication, especially the use personal distance to understand how people define or relate themselves with respect to others. To understand this difference, he described four different zones people tend to create around others. These are dependent on their relationships, and how people react when these zones are invaded. The zones of personal space include: *intimate distance*, *personal distance*, *social distance*, and *public distance*. *Intimate* distance is up to one and a half feet. This space is typically reserved for very few social contacts, such as intimate partners, and parents and children. *Personal* distance is further than the intimate distance but up to 4 ft. This space is generally reserved for friends. *Social* distance is from four to 12 ft, usually observed in a formal business settings such as a meeting between doctor and patient. *Public* distance is beyond 12 ft and reserved for those who perform to an audience. Interestingly, when these distances are not respected, people feel discomfort and may try to regain their space by moving away or creating a boundary (e.g. using books or a bag while sitting on a bench in a park).

Harold Garfinkel developed a perspective that refers to the study of how people make sense of what others say and do in the course of day-to-day social interaction. This perspective is referred to as **ethnomethodology** and is formally defined as "the study of professional and nonprofessional methods through which social order is produced" (Lewis-Beck et al. 2004). It is a fascinating approach that allows us to reveal the lengths to which people will go to maintain norms. It also clearly shows us how often we regularly engage in norm maintenance ourselves. A relatively common and fun class experiment in introduction to sociology is to go out and "break norms" then observe as people attempt to regain normalcy. Students conducting these experiments have engaged in a range of behaviors including standing to face people in an elevator (rather than standing toward the elevator door), dancing in a restaurant while having breakfast, or standing on people's toes in line at the grocery store. In response, these students got reactions ranging from the very mild (strange looks) to the more extreme (physical advances), which they observed and detailed. The important point of these activities is to reveal how important it is, and how common, to maintain norms and the lengths to which people will go to do so. Garfinkel thus argued that the study of micro- interaction is critical to understand shared cultural assumptions and unstated knowledge carried out in every day interaction.

3.4 Contemporary Research on Social Interaction

Drawing from ethnomethodology, conversation analysis examines details of daily conversations to reveal organizational principles in the conversations (usually assumed) and how they may contribute to the production and reproduction of the social order. Imagine a situation where a homeless man on the street tries to engage in a conversation with a young woman walking by. He may start with friendly openings, such as "hey, pretty" and "how you doin?" to her, but the woman may either give him a short answer by saying "hi" or just ignore him. Even when he may attempt to elicit further responses from the woman, she may walk away. On the surface, the fact that the woman ignored him may be seen as rude, or perhaps unusual as that is not how people usually interact with each other. However, this unwanted interaction is tied to the gender hierarchy and social stratification in our society. For example, men may feel privileged to make advances toward a young women who, on the other hand, may be physically vulnerable. Similarly, there is a clear difference in class status between the two individuals that leads to a greater likelihood that the woman will ignore the man given his homeless status.

Let's take another situation that may also seem purely micro-level on its face: In New York City, a taxi driver tries to make a small talk with a passenger who happens to be Asian.

Driver: "where you from?"
Passenger: "I am from New York."
Driver: "I mean, where you originally from? Are you Chinese?"
Passenger: "What?"

From this situation, you can see that the driver just assumed that the Asian passenger is an immigrant, perhaps from China. Through the use of conversation analysis we may links micro-level interactions between individuals to a broader social context. The link between micro- and macro- sociology allows us to better understand these interactions and individuals' social behaviors.

3.4.1 Doctor-Patient Interaction

Theories of social interaction are also useful in medical sociology. Medical treatment usually begins with a conversation between a medical provider and a patient. The effective interaction of a doctor with a patient is extremely important as the information gathered from the interaction guides subsequent treatments. As such, it is important to understand how the various roles occupied by each and the factors that have shaped their identities, can lead to relatively more or fewer positive encounters in a health setting.

3.4.2 Sick Role

In order to understand doctor-patient interaction, it is important to review the concept of the *sick role* that Talcott Parsons introduced. First, let's review the definition of health. According to the World Health Organization (WHO), health is defined broadly as a 'state of complete physical mental, and social well-being and not merely the absence of disease or infirmity' (World Health Organization 2006). Accordingly, the sick role is defined as the established expectations associated with illness and how a person should act if they are sick or perceived as sick or deviant. We learn how we should behave in this sick role through the process of socialization. Perhaps in your family, being sick meant you were babied and someone catered to your needs. This understanding is culturally based and varies not only within families but across groups. As a society we have a shared understanding of acceptable behavior in accordance with the sick role and this is reflected in work policies that provide for time off and long-term disability pay.

Parsons conceived of health as a valued commodity that would allow individuals to effectively perform their social roles (Parsons 1951). According to this theory, illness indicates the individual's inability to fully function in accordance with their social roles. Parsons used the term, *sick role*, to refer to the status that individuals assume when they experience illness (and therefore cannot fully function as a part of the society). Parsons further specified the sick role with four features: including two rights and two obligations. Based on the two rights, individuals with illness can claim: (1) that they cannot perform their social roles to maintain the society functioning; and (2) that the illness is one to blame. For the two responsibilities, those with illness are expected: (1) to *want* to get well; and (2) actively to *seek* professional help and to *cooperate* with the healthcare provider. Thus, we as a society base our support of someone who is sick on some of the decisions they make and our perceptions about their willingness to recover.

The concept of the sick role by Parsons has received critiques. First, the categorization of those with illness vs. those without it is too simple to characterize the complex experiences among individuals when they have illness. Second, Parsons ignores the fact that people with an illness can still function, as he treated illness as reflecting incapacity to function once they have an illness. Third, while the concept of the sick role works for those with acute disease, it does not apply for those with chronic health conditions that require care and treatment for a long period. Finally, Parsons assumed that the responsibility of the patient is passive, willingly cooperating with the care provider to get well. However, in reality, the roles of patients are crucial in the treatment process. They are incorporated in every aspect from initiating the process, to diagnosing of disease, exploring treatment options, deciding on treatment method(s), and treating the disease (Annandale 2014). Despite these critiques, his concept served to invite sociologists to further discussion about social model of illness and doctor-patient relationship.

In the Health Setting. Recent research has increasingly uncovered the importance of patient activation, a term which refers to empowerment of patients to take an active role in their health and its role on improved health outcomes. Health professionals should strive to encourage patient activation when possible and recognize that there may be distinct differences in the level of patient activation observed across racial, ethnic, and gender groups, among others.

3.4.3 Three Models for Doctor-Patient Interaction

Since Parsons introduced the concept of the sick role it has been expanded with respect to the rights and obligations of health care providers. Subsequent research elaborates the social models for the doctor-patient relationship by adding two additional concepts relevant to specific situations. The three models are: (1) the activity-passivity model; (2) the guidance-cooperation model; and (3) the mutual participation model (Szasz and Hollander 1956). In the **activity-passivity model**, the doctor is totally active while the patient is totally passive. This model applies in an emergency room setting where the patient is seriously ill, and thus not able to communicate with the doctor. The doctor is expected to make treatment decisions for the patient, and the patient makes little contribution to the interaction with the doctor. The second model, the **guidance-cooperation model**, is the most common in the doctor-patient interactions, and applies when the patient has an acute health condition, such as an infectious illness. In this model, the doctor still makes treatment decisions. However, the doctor offers guidance to the patient first, and the patient who suffers from the illness cooperates with the doctor by following the doctor's guidance. Third, the **mutual participation model** applies when the doctor and the patient participate in the interactions equally. This model occurs most often with the management of chronic illness, such as diabetes or heart disease in which the doctor's role is mostly to manage the pain and to help the patient find the best treatment options. The patient often adjusts their own lifestyle and takes medication according to what the doctor recommends and suggests. But, the treatment process requires mutual and active participations from both sides.

Hopefully, it is clear that power dynamics differ across these models. For example, doctors' power is the greatest in the situations when patients are completely incapacitated by coma or stroke, which is often the case for the activity-passivity model. Importantly, the power dynamics within these models may differ depending on several factors. According to Freidson (1970), a doctor's power also increases when they have cultural authority. This means that there are some situations in which their status as a doctor is highly important and recognized as such by the patient. Physicians may use their culturally accepted authority to convince patients whether and what treatments patient should receive. It is important to recognize this authority and the fact that some groups may be more or less submissive in a treatment setting. The second factor is the doctors' economic independence. For example, a doctor's power is greater among those working in group practices compared to those who practice at individual clinics. Finally, doctors' power is greater with patients whose primary language is different from the doctors,' and with patients who have different cultural background and have lower social status (Street 1991).

Weitz (2007) also explored how doctors establish and maintain their authority over patients from existing studies using conversation analysis (e.g. Fisher 1986; Katz 1984; Mishler 1990; Waitzkin 1991; West 1984). From this literature, Weitz (2007) identified several patterns found in the conversations between doctors and patients during their meetings. First, conversations between doctors and patients typically start when the doctor initiates it by asking questions of the patient. These questions are usually closed-ended rather than open-ended. Through the use of closed-ended questions, patients are expected to stay on the topic that doctors are interested in, rather than being encouraged to raise a new topic that patients may want to discuss with their doctor. Second, when patients answer questions from doctors, doctors have been shown to interrupt patients more often than patients interrupt doctors. Third, when patients ask questions, doctors often give general answers rather than specific information pertaining to the question as it was asked. This often leaves patients confused or unclear on the issue that they raised. Lastly, doctors introduce themselves with a professional title (i.e. Dr.) and expect patients to refer to them by this title, while they often refer to patients by first name.

3.4.4 Potential Threats to Doctor-Patient Interaction

From the above, there is evidence that doctors often dominate conversations with patients by engaging in several tactics to control the topics that are discussed. Additional threats may further harm the effectiveness of the doctor-patient interaction, and these relate to the characteristics of patients. Specifically, interactions may be harmed when there are socioeconomic status, gender, and cultural differences between doctors and patients.

With respect to the socioeconomic status of patients, lower-class patients are more likely to take a passive role when interacting with doctors. Comparatively, middle and upper class patients tend to be more consumer-oriented and active in conversations with doctors (Cockerham et al. 1986). As a result, lower status patients are more likely to be less informed about their treatment options, procedures, and consequences of the treatments.

Gender can also influence the interactions between doctors and patients. For instance, male doctors may lack sensitivity to female patients when discussing issues related to pregnancy, childbirth, and breast cancer. Combined with a higher proportion of females belonging to lower social status groups, opinions and circumstances of female patients regarding treatment options may not be well considered. In comparison, female physicians are often perceived as less of an authority figure than male doctors (West 1984). Accordingly, patients may not take guidance from female doctors for treatment very seriously.

Finally, doctor and patient interaction may also be influenced by cultural differences, which are particularly important in the current US society, which is highly diverse and where a substantial proportion of the population consists of immigrants. Importantly, immigrants from different cultural backgrounds may have different meanings associated with illness and thus respond to illness differently. Furthermore, doctors cannot assume that questions asked in English will have the same meaning to those who are from different culture, especially those with limited English proficiency.

Key Terms

- **Self-Identity**: a definition of individual personality and self-image, formulated through the ongoing process of self-development through interactions between ourselves and the work around us over the life course
- **Transgender**: individuals whose gender identity is not align with sex assigned at birth
- **Cisgender**: individuals whose gender identity is align with sex assigned at birth
- **Prejudice**: a generalization about an entire category of people based on little or no direct evidence
- **Stereotype**: a description applied to every person in a social group based on prejudice about the group
- **Stereotype Threat**: a situational predicament where people feel at risk of conforming to existing stereotypes against the social group of which they are members
- **Social Identity**: social characteristics of an individual, in terms of gender, race/ethnicity and social roles, which place that individual in related to others who share the same attributes
- **Dramaturgical Approach**: a theatrical setting used to analyze human behaviors
- **Impression Management**: preparation for the presentation of one's social role on a stage
- **Personal Space**: personal distance on how people define or relate themselves with respect to others
- **Ethnomethodology**: the study of professional of nonprofessional methods through which social order is produced
- **Conversation Analysis**: an analytical approach that examines details of daily conversations to reveal organizational principles in the conversation and how they may contribute to the production and reproduction of the social order
- **Sick Role**: the status that individuals assume when they experience illness and cannot fully function as a part of the society
- **Three Models for the Doctor and Patient Relationship**
  - **Activity-passivity model**: the doctor is totally active while the patient is totally passive
  - **Guidance-cooperation model**: the doctor offers guidance to the patient first and the patient cooperates with the doctor
  - **Mutual participation model**: the doctor and the patient participate in the interactions equally

Activities and Discussion Questions

In June 2017, the State of Oregon became the first state to recognize non-binary people, those who identify themselves neither male nor female, on their driver's licenses. The State of California joined Oregon as the senate passed the bill to allow their residents to be non-gender binary, and a similar bill has been introduced in New York and the District of Columbia.

Form a group with one or two additional members for the following activities.

Activity 1. Identify what impacts this change in gender categorization might make among individuals, in terms of gender identity development process.

Activity 2. Think of any potential health related issues that those who identify as gender non-binary, whose pronoun is "they," might experience, and discuss how health professionals might respond to their needs.

Discussion Question 1. Identify important factors that shape self-identity and think of ways how self-identity may affect social behaviors.

Discussion Question 2. How do doctors achieve and maintain professionalism while interacting with patients?

Discussion Question 3. What is cultural competence? Why is it important and what possible consequences are expected when it is ignored?

Study Questions

1. **Define the terms: self-identity and social identity.**
2. **How does gender, race, and culture influence interactions?**
3. **What factors have been shown to influence the power dynamics between patients and providers?**

***Example Exam Question:** "Anxious about an illness, a non-native English speaker asks their doctor about some related symptoms. The doctor replies with a general response, and because of cultural differences, the patient does not ask any more questions. Which concept would be most relevant for explaining this miscommunication?

A. Power and status differentials
B. Impression management
C. Social support
D. The sick role"

*The above example is an author created question, please refer to *The Official Guide to the MCAT Exam*, 4th Edition (AAMC 2015) for additional sample questions and information on the entrance exam.

References

Annandale, E. (2014). *The sociology of health and medicine: A critical introduction* (2nd ed.). Malden: Polity Press.

Association of American Medical Colleges (AAMC). (2012). *Preview guide for the MCAT 2015 exam* (2nd ed.). www.aamc.org/MCAT2015

Association of American Medical Colleges (AAMC). (2015). *The official guide to the MCAT exam* (MCAT 2015) (4th ed.). Washington, DC: The Association of American Medical Colleges.
Bussey, K. (2011). Gender Identity Development. In S. J. Schwartz, K. Luyckx, & V. L. Vignoles (Eds.), *Handbook of identity theory and research*. New York City: Springer.
Cockerham, W. C., Lueschen, G., Kunz, G., & Spaeth, J. L. (1986). Social stratification and self-Management of Health. *Journal of Health and Social Behavior, 27*, 1–14.
Dovidio, J. F., & Gaertner, S. L. (2010). Intergroup bias. In S. T. Fiske, D. T. Gilbert, & G. Lindzey (Eds.), *The handbook of social psychology* (Vol. 2, 5th ed.). New York City: Wiley.
Featherman, D. L. (1983). *The life-span perspective in social science research*. Center for Demography and Ecology Working Paper, 81–85.
Fisher, S. (1986). *In the Patient's best interest: Women and the politics of medical decisions*. New Brunswick: Rutgers University Press.
Flores, A. R., Herman, J. L., Gates, G. J., & Brown, T. N. T. (2016). *How many adults identify as transgender in the United States*. Los Angeles: The Williams Institute.
Fordham, S., & Ogbu, J. U. (1986). Black students' school success: Coping with the burden of acting white. *The Urban Review, 18*(3), 176–206.
Freidson, E. (1970). *Professional dominance*. Chicago: Aldine.
Gainor, K. A. (2000). Including transgender issues in lesbian, gay, and bisexual psychology: Implications for clinical practice and training. In B. Greene & G. L. Croom (Eds.), *Education, research, and practice in lesbian, gay, bisexual, and transgendered psychology: A resource manual*. Thousand Oaks: Sage.
Giddens, A., Duneier, M., Appelbaum, R. P., & Carr, D. (2016). *Introduction to sociology (10th Ed)*. New York City: W.W. Norton & Company.
Hegewisch, A., Liepmann, H., Hayes, J., & Hartmann, H. (2010). *Separate and not equal? Gender segregation in the labor market and the gender wage gap*. Washington, DC: The Institute for Women's Policy Research.
Katz, J. (1984). *The silent world of doctor and patient*. New York City: Free Press.
Lewis-Beck, M. S., Bryman, A., & Liao, T. F. (Eds.). (2004). *The Sage encyclopedia of social science research methods* (3rd ed.). Thousand Oaks: Sage.
Leaper, C. (2002). Parenting girls and boys. In M. H. Bornstein (Ed.), *Handbook of parenting (2nd Ed), volume 1 children and parenting*. Mahwah: Lawrence Erlbaum Associates.
McGarty, C., Yzerbyt, V. Y., & Spears, R. (2002). Social, cultural and cognitive factors in stereotype formation. In *In Stereotypes as Explanations: The Formation of Meaningful Beliefs about Social Groups*. Cambridge: Cambridge University Press.
Mishler, E. G. (1990). The struggle between the voice of medicine and the voice of the Lifeworld. In P. Conrad & R. Kern (Eds.), *The sociology of health and illness: Critical perspectives* (pp. 295–307). New York: St. Martin's Press.
Morin, R. (2015, August 19). *Exploring racial bias among biracial and single-race adults: The IAT*. Pew Research Center, Washington, DC.
Parsons, T. (1951). *The social system*. New York City: Free Press.
Schilt, K., & Westbook, L. (2009). gender Normals, transgender people, and the social maintenance of heterosexuality. *Gender & Society, 23*(4), 440–464.
Steele, C. M., & Aronson, J. (1995). Stereotype threat and the intellectual test performance of African Americans. *Journal of Personality and Social Psychology, 69*(5), 797–811.
Street, R. (1991). Information giving in medical consultations: The influence of patients' communicative styles and personal characteristics. *Social Science & Medicine, 32*, 541–548.
Szasz, T. S., & Hollander, M. H. (1956). A contribution to the philosophy of medicine. *Archives of Internal Medicine, 97*, 585–592.
Waitzkin, H. (1991). *The politics of medical encounters*. New Haven: Yale University Press.
Weitz, R. (2007). *The sociology of health, illness, and health care*. Belmont: Thomson Higher Education.
West, C. (1984). *Routine complications: Troubles with talk between doctors and patients*. Bloomington: Indiana University Press.
West, C., & Zimmerman, D. H. (1987). Doing Gender. *Gender and Society, 1*(2), 125–151.
World Health Organization. (2006). *Constitution of the World Health Organization – Basic Documents* (45th Ed), retrieved from the website at http://www.who.int/governance/eb/who_constitution_en.pdf

Chapter 4
Social Interaction, Socialization, and Group Influence

Part 1: Social Interactions and Socialization: will discuss the ways we interact with each other, types of communication, and the socialization process

Part 2: Group Influence and Dynamics: will discuss the distinction between PSY and SOC (outside influences versus inner), sociologically define groups, and consider the micro- and macro-level study of groups

Objectives

- Understand how social processes influence human behavior and identity
- Review basic sociological concepts related to social interaction, socialization, and groups
- Link social interaction/support (and isolation) to health outcomes

Foundational Concept 7

"*Biological, psychological, and sociocultural factors influence behavior and behavior change…*

Human behavior is complex and often surprising, differing across individuals in the same situation and within an individual across different situations. A full understanding of human behavior requires knowledge of the interplay between psychological, socio-cultural, and biological factors that are related to behavior. This interplay has important implications for the way we behave and the likelihood of behavior change. Foundational Concept 7 focuses on individual and social determinants of behavior and behavior change" (AAMC 2015: 99).

Category 7B (social processes that influence human behavior) focuses on how social factors, such as groups and culture, affect behavior.

(continued)

G. Garcia-Alexander et al., *Social Foundations of Behavior for the Health Sciences*,
DOI 10.1007/978-3-319-64950-4_4

Foundational Concept 8

"*Psychological, socio-cultural, and biological factors influence the way we think about ourselves and others...*

Human beings are social by nature. Though the sentiment is simple, the actions and processes underlying and shaping our social interactions are not" (AAMC 2012: 108).

Category 8C (social interactions) focuses on the actions and processes underlying social interactions.

4.1 Sociocultural Impacts on Behavior and Health

Research has shown that behaviors, and more specifically, health-related behaviors vary from one group to another, and that they are linked to various health outcomes. The strength, quantity, and quality of our social ties with others also play a role in our overall health, and sociologists have studied the impacts of *social support* and *isolation*. The pathways connecting social bonds and behavior patterns to disease are complex, and a general understanding of the factors that influence these things is necessary for the development of a medical vocabulary. Training in such factors will better equip students to make informed decisions and recommendations related to the promotion of healthy behaviors and interventions.

Additionally, it is important to recognize how we think about ourselves and others. We learn how to be members of society through the socialization process. This process has an important impact on our development and understanding of social situations. Further, the ways in which we interact with others are influenced by our understanding of the social world; and it is necessary to recognize these influences in order to be able to work well with patients.

An entire body of research has developed around the concept of *patient-provider interactions* and its impacts. Generally, the research in this area indicates that the quality of the relationship between doctors and their patients, along with the nature of the interaction itself, has an important and measureable impact on patients' health behaviors and outcomes. Factors that influence these interactions include such things as language barriers, whether the patient and provider belong to the same racial/ethnic group, whether accommodations are made in accordance with patient needs, and the level of cultural competency of the provider. Findings from this field indicate that members of racial/ethnic minority and low-income groups are significantly more likely to report poor communication with health providers (AHRQ 2016). In addition, stereotyping and implicit bias on the part of physicians has been shown to lead to disparities in treatment (Dovidio et al. 2008). However, a patient-centered approach that encompasses compassion, empathy, and responsiveness to the needs/values/preferences of individual patients has been shown to improve health status (Stewart et al. 2000), lessen symptom burden, encourage compliance with treatment (Haskard Zolnierek and DiMatteo 2009), and reduce misdiagnosing. Thus, becoming aware of the importance of interpersonal interactions and implicit biases that may hinder the development of quality care is of great importance to those in the health profession.

4.2 A Sociological Understanding of Interactions, Behavior, and Socialization

4.2.1 Social Interaction and Norms

It is important to begin with the understanding that sociology differs from orientations (like psychology and biology) which locate the nexus for behavior and behavioral change within the individual. In contrast, sociologists are careful to focus on the influence of external factors on decision-making and behavior. Accordingly, we concentrate on how social norms and group contexts play a role in determining and governing our behavior. **Social norms** refer to the principles or rules of social life that were are expected to observe. These will vary by culture and over time. Social norms are transmitted via **social interaction** (behavior between two or more people that is given meaning). During social interactions, social cues are transmitted through language (sociologists consider language a symbol), i.e. verbal communication; as well as facial expressions, body language, pitch and tone of voice, and other forms of **non-verbal communication**. These messages or cues are perceived and interpreted by those engaged in social interactions and inform our understanding of the world. In addition, (and as discussed in an earlier chapter on identity) they play a key role in the development of our identity, or who we become. Accordingly, we are constantly engaged in social interactions that shape our current and future behavior. In a health context, non-verbal communication is important as it may communicate various messages to those we interact with. Non-verbal communication has been shown to affect the quality of the patient-provider relationship and may act as a medium through which subtle, or aversive, racism is transmitted. Thus, racial minorities have been shown to perceive non-verbal cues of prejudice through eye contact (or lack thereof), markers of anxiety (rapid blinking), and other friendliness cues (Dovidio et al. 2008). These non-verbal messages can potentially harm the patient encounter and ultimately may contribute to health disparities observed for some minority groups.

In today's society, the role of non-verbal communication can also be considered in the context of online exchanges. Increasingly, more attention has been given to the rise in internet usage and online social interaction. This has had major impacts on people's social relationships and the ways in which they communicate with one another. Amazingly, the percentage of adults using social networking sites increased from 8% in 2005 to 76% in 2015 (PEW Research Center 2016). Figure 4.1 depicts the level of social media usage among various age groups. Clear differences emerge on the basis of age with 90% of those 18–29 reporting social media use in 2013.

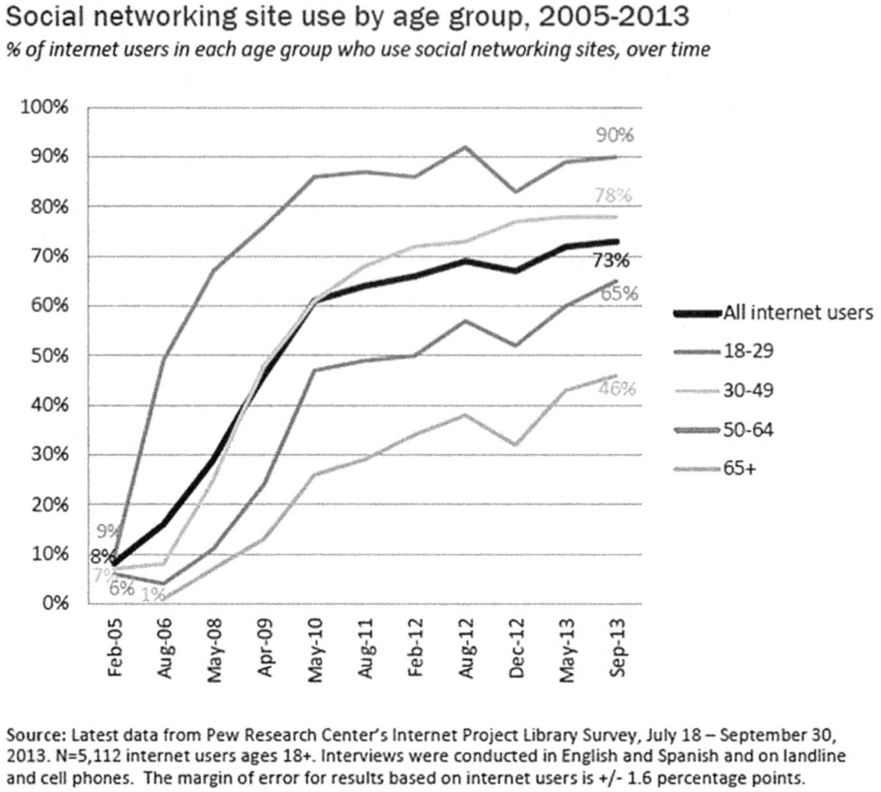

Fig. 4.1 Social networking site usage by age group

Such widespread use of social media and internet has led to increased questions surrounding its impacts on socialization as it has the potential to fundamentally alter social interactions and their meanings. Some argue increased online interaction will lead to social isolation and an inability to engage in deep, meaningful relationships. Others argue that the widespread social media/internet usage will enhance social interactions and allow people to expand their networks. No clear consensus exists on the ultimate impacts of increased online interaction; however, it will be important to consider the opportunities and potential for negative impacts of such changes in a health setting.

4.2.2 Social Networks

Sociologists have long-studied **social networks**, or the ways we're connected to each other, to better understand social behavior. Formally, social networks refer to the web of social relationships surrounding a person, ranging from weak to strong.

The strength of these ties is indicated by a combination of time spent, emotional intensity, intimacy, and reciprocation present in interpersonal relations (Granovetter 1973). Social network theory tells us that social actors who have central positions networks have greater access to power and resources as a result of their web of connections. In a famous study conducted by Mark S. Granovetter, *The Strength of Weak Ties* (1973), he differentiated strong ties (those with people we're close to, e.g. family and friends) from weak ties (those with people we consider acquaintances) to illustrate how our network of connections operates in daily life. Ironically, he showed that strong ties were less important than weak ties in how people got jobs. This may be counterintuitive since you might expect that the people you are closest to/have the strongest connections with would be more likely to help you get a job. But, this research showed that the networks people are connected to through weak ties were broader and offered greater access to opportunities. In fact, most people report getting a job through a weak tie since this widens the web of opportunities.

In terms of how this research connects to online social networks, it's important to note how this concept applies. Social networking sites like Facebook and Twitter allow us to be connected to a great many people who are our "friends" or followers. These different types of social media allow people who are widely distributed (geographically) to be connected to one another. Formally, these would be considered weak ties. But, it's argued that these ties are much weaker than those described in the studies mentioned above (Ritzer and Ryan 2010). Accordingly, the research in this area indicates less agreement about how these online connections may be harnessed. One position suggests that social media usage has expanded our connections to others and increased their diversity (Hampton et al. 2011). It's also argued that greater use of social media leads to more opportunities to develop local ties. An alternate position is that widespread social media use has led to smaller networks that are less diverse (McPherson et al. 2006). It is further argued that social media has allowed us to replace face-to-face interactions with online forms.

In the Health Setting: Sociologists are further interested in how increased use of social networking sites and online engagement may contribute to feelings of social isolation or social support. **Social isolation** refers to a lack of social relationships while **social support** refers to the willingness of those in one's social networks to provide financial, informational, or emotional support (Berkman 2000; Smith and Christakis 2008; Thoits 1995). This is especially relevant in the health field as these concepts have been shown to impact well-being. For example, a number of studies have shown that people who are socially isolated have a greater mortality risk than those who have more robust social connections (House et al. 1988). On the other hand, those with better social relationships have improved health outcomes. This has been shown to be the case because our social ties influence our health habits positively, provide social support and meaning, and reduce stress responses (Umberson and Montez 2010).

On the other hand, social relationships may produce stress and/or promote unhealthy habits or health risks. As the use of social networking continues to grow, further research will be needed to determine how this form of interaction may hinder or promote health and well-being. High levels of online interaction will also impact the nature of exchanges between those in the healthcare setting and patients. For example, a number of initiatives have begun to support the development of alternate modes of delivery of care for various populations. Such modes include: tele-health services, app-based/on-demand doctor visits, and online consultations and sessions.

4.2.3 Socialization

We learn the informal and formal rules of behavior through a process called **socialization**. This is a lifelong process that begins with the development of basic social skills, the formation of our core identity, and continues on throughout the life course to teach us the expectations of society. Importantly, we should understand that there are different perspectives on how we develop our identities. A sociological perspective recognizes the importance of culture and our social environment on shaping human behavior. In contrast, biological determinism describes the perspective that our biology fully explains our patterns of behavior. This debate can broadly be characterized as a *nature* (biological determinism) vs. *nurture* (social determinism) debate (for more information, see Further Thought). Sociologists do not necessarily argue that there is no impact of biology, but they do focus on the importance of the social learning process and the amount of time humans spend instilling the values and roles of our culture. In other words, they try to understand how biology and social learning intersect. To demonstrate the importance of the socialization process, sociologists often look to instances of social isolation. In these cases, individuals experienced extreme isolation or a lack of contact in their early years. Examples include work conducted by Spitz (1945) in which he compared infants raised in a nursery for children of women in prison to those in an orphanage. For the most part these settings were very similar – they both provided clean environments and attention to basic human needs. But, the major difference between these two settings was that in the nursery, the children were regularly exposed to attendants and visitors. In the orphanage, there was little human contact except for feedings or changing. While the babies in the nurseries did not suffer from many emotional or physical issues, the ones in the orphanage developed emotional and physical problems (some of which led to death). These problems were reduced once interaction was increased. Another extreme example is that of "Genie", a young girl who was abused and kept severely isolated until she was thirteen years old. She did not interact with people and was not able to develop language skills. Once her case was discovered, a team of scientists worked with her to encourage development, and she ultimately was able to develop basic social skills and nonverbal communication. But, she was never able to fully acquire a language (see links for more information). These cases are especially important to sociologists because they have shown us that the experience of bonding and early interaction with other humans is crucial to the development of normal intelligence, the ability to be social, and the ability to internalize and follow societal norms.

Box 4.1: Further Thought
Nature vs. Nurture (studies involving twins): Are we destined to become/do/be [fill in the blank] on the basis of our biological makeup? Or, are we the product of lifelong learning? To better understand how to answer this question we can consider studies that examine twins in an attempt to separate the role of genetics and environment. The ideal way to examine this would be to examine identical twins separated at birth, but because those cases are so rare, scholars have studied identical twins in comparison to fraternal twins. In these studies, it has been argued that genetics, i.e. nature, do seem to play an important role in development. For example, hyperactivity and reading disability appear to be attributable to genetic factors (Guo 2005). However, the environment also plays a role in various outcomes (though the effect is smaller in traditional twin studies). Importantly, it is becoming increasingly recognized that genes interact with environment, and social scientists can help to understand that process. What studies of twins tell us is that some traits are hereditary – but they are often subject to social influence.

Those who we surrounded and interact with play a key role in transmitting the norms and expectations of the society into which we are born. Thus, socialization is different on the basis of such things as gender, race or ethnicity, class, religion and so on. As mentioned above, sociologists focus on the external influences (our family, friends, teachers, etc.) that contribute to the socialization process as opposed to focusing on inherent traits that produce variations in human behavior. For more information see Box 4.1 (Further Thought).

We can also differentiate between early socialization, primary; and later socialization, secondary. *Primary* socialization refers to the earliest phase of socialization (infancy and childhood) in which we learn basic social skills and start to develop our identities. This can also be thought of as the first socialization, through which we become members of society (Appelrouth and Edles 2012). A number of theories of child development have emerged to explain this process, some of which come from a sub-field of sociology, social psychology. An important contributor to this area was George H. Mead, who described the process by which we pass through various stages and undergo the development of self. He identified important concepts including the "I", which represents our un-socialized self/infant, the "me" which represents our socialized self, and the "generalized other", which refers to the general values of our culture. He focused on the idea that infants/children learn develop by imitating those around them and engaging in games. For example, when children "play house" they are imitating the behavior of adults around them in preparation for that phase in their own lives. Early on, we imitate those who are closest to us (for instance, our family members), and as we engage and interact with more people we start to internalize the values and expectations of society and develop a sense of self. Formally, self-awareness develops when we can differentiate between the "I′ and the "me". *Secondary socialization* takes place in childhood and continues on into maturity. It can also be thought of as a phase of socialization that brings the already socialized individual into new facets of society, and it is often acquired by choice as one prepares for new stages in life. As mentioned before, socialization is a lifelong process that is continually reinforced through social interaction.

Importantly, socialization also serves as a social control mechanism. What this means is that we are trained to internalize our culture's definition of what is acceptable, and we use sanctions to regulate interactions. This encourages conformity and discourages deviance. As we accept norms, we behave accordingly. We also reinforce the norms and expectations of society as we transmit them on to others. Socialization produces conforming members of society through a lifelong process of receiving rewards (positive sanctions) when we conform, and punishments (negative sanctions) when we do not. These rewards and punishments can range from very subtle to overt coercion in accordance with the severity of the violation. For example, if a person cuts in line at the grocery store, they might get a dirty look or be told to go to the back of the line. This is a relatively minor sanction for "breaking the rules" or violating a norm. On the other hand, one might be sent to prison for many years for a serious violation such as physical assault or homicide.

We are socialized by various different individuals, groups, and social contexts. Those that have a direct impact on our self-concept, attitudes, behavior, and orientations to the world are known as **agents of socialization**. Examples of such agents include the family, schools, the media, peers, religion, and sports, among others. The family is typically our first and most important agent of primary socialization. Family structures may vary from one culture to another and within cultures. Here in the U.S., the dominant form is known as the nuclear family. This refers to a family unit that is comprised of an adult parent(s) and their dependent children. Parents transmit cultural/social norms with respect to appropriate behavior, learning skills, a sense of right and wrong, and so on. As would be expected, these values and messages may vary largely from one family to the next. For example, some families may place a great deal of emphasis on education or achievement while others may place little to no emphasis on this goal.

Over time, the influence of the family diminishes as agents including peer and schools come to serve as sources of socialization. Schools in particular transmit traditional educational information, but they also serve as an important source of information on what is known as the "hidden curriculum". This refers to the informal rules of behavior that apply in the classroom, i.e. learning to be on time, sitting quietly for extended periods, raising your hand to ask a question, and so on. Some interesting research in this area has shown that these messages vary on the basis of social class. In a well-known study, different schools were compared in terms of the "hidden curriculum". It was found that in working class schools, children were evaluated in terms of whether they followed the correct steps (rather than whether the answer was correct) and a more directive style was used. In middle class schools, following directions and getting the right answers was stressed, along with thinking through the work. In affluent schools, students were encouraged to work independently and be creative, and children have a say in or negotiate the work to be done. These different styles of education have a clear socializing influence with working and middle class students being taught to conform and follow rules and upper class students being trained to be creative and assume leadership (Anyon 1980). Peer groups are another source of socialization that becomes increasingly important over the life course. Thus, the relationships we develop with people who are similar in age will impact our views and shape our behaviors. Finally, the media has become an increasingly important agent of socialization that impacts our attitudes and beliefs.

Socialization is further patterned according to **social roles**. These are the socially defined expectations that a person in a given social position, or **status**, follows. Through the process of socialization, we learn how to behave appropriately and in line with what others expect of us on the basis of the roles we occupy. For example, we may be a friend, a daughter, a teacher, a student, or many other things, and we adjust our behavior to reflect the role we are playing. An influential sociologist, Erving Goffman, posited that social life can be thought of as a series of performances that one takes on in various settings and situations (we are all social actors). Thus, he identified **role performance**, which refers to "all the activity of a given participant on a given occasion which serves to influence in any way any of the other participants" (1959; 15); while **impression management** refers to the conscious manipulation of others' perceptions. Accordingly, we may choose to emphasize certain behaviors that we consider to be reflective of a given role, while we suppress/avoid behaviors that are at odds with a given impression. So, in a way, we are manipulating others into seeing us in a particular way. Take for example a job interview – people dress in a specific way, avoid topics/subjects that may make them appear less employable, redefine past situations to give the impression that certain skills are present and so on.

Gender or sex role socialization refers to the ongoing process through which individuals learn to take on the acceptable behaviors and expectations for males and females. This differential process has little to do with biology and much more to do with society's expectations for what it means to be female, i.e. feminine, and male, i.e. masculine. Dominant/mainstream messages about masculinity define it as assertive, aggressive, strong, and heterosexual (Connell 1987). In contrast femininity refers to passivity, nurturing, caring, and subordinate (Connell 1987). However, society plays a tremendous role in defining these concepts, and messages about sex roles are transmitted continuously via the family, our peers, the media, religious organizations, and so on. For example, studies have shown that boys and girls are handled differently in infancy (male infants are handled more roughly while female infants are handled more gently), boys and girls are dressed in different colors, given different toys to play with, and so on. Interesting research in this area has looked at children's books to examine how messages about gender are transmitted very early on. The earliest research indicated that the stereotypical female and male traits were heavily portrayed in children's books. Thus, male characters were shown as competent and achievement oriented while females were nearly invisible or depicted as passive followers (Weitzman et al. 1972). More recent studies have shown that these disparities continue to be reflected and send strong messages about what it means to be male or female.

In the Health Setting: Researchers have found consistent differences in how men and women use health care services. For example, in the U.S. women are much more likely to use preventive care while men are more likely to use the E.R. Some of this could be explained by women's needs for reproductive services. However, sex role socialization plays a greater role in these behavioral differences. Research has shown us that women have been socialized to be more aware of symptoms. Comparatively, masculinity is often noted as an explanation for delayed help-seeking among men. For a review of the literature on this topic see Galdas et al. 2005 (also see Andersen 1995 and Pescosolido 1992 in *Resources, Links, and Recommended Readings* section).

Doing gender refers to the idea that we act in accordance with gender roles as well as perceive others' behaviors in line with the expectations we have learned about gender roles (West and Zimmerman 1987). In other words, we construct differences on the basis of social definitions and then use those definitions to argue there are "real differences" between sexes. This is an ongoing process that occurs during social interactions. Increasingly, scholars in this area have considered the problematic nature of focusing on and reinforcing the notion of two mutually exclusive categories of gender. Scholars such as Judith Butler and Patricia Hill Collins have questioned some feminists' use of traditional categories that serve to reinforce sexism. Certainly the separation of the biological sex from the social gender was an achievement, but Butler challenges this further by contending that gender is by no means fixed and is only sustained by gender performativity (1991). In other words, binary categories are reinforced by the process of *doing gender*, whereby we accept and confirm the notion of two genders.

Butler is also well-known for the development of queer theory. Prior to the 1990s, the term queer had negative connotations. But, scholars in this area (including Butler) worked to reclaim the term and its meaning by suggesting that all sexual identities and categories are social constructs. In today's society, this is reflected by much more fluid ideas about gender identity and sexual orientation, which have come to achieve much greater acceptance (see GLAAD's report on acceptance in America at: http://www.glaad.org/files/aa/2017_GLAAD_Accelerating_Acceptance.pdf). As an example, in 2014 Facebook rolled out a list of 58 gender options for users to choose from. These included such categories as: agender, bigender, cisgender, among others. For a full list of categories see: http://abcnews.go.com/blogs/headlines/2014/02/heres-a-list-of-58-gender-options-for-facebook-users/.

4.3 Groups and Organizations

4.3.1 Groups

Sociologists study how and why we come together and form groups for various purposes. We all belong to all sorts of different groups such as our families, peer groups, sports teams, co-workers, professional associations, and so on. **Groups** can be defined as a collection of individuals who: (1) interact with one another, (2) share goals and norms, and (3) have a subjective awareness of themselves as a "we". Some examples of groups include our families, peer groups, and professional associations. From a sociological standpoint, groups can be differentiated from social aggregates, which are collections of people who may or may not interact, but do not have a shared sense of belonging with one another. As an example, those in a movie audience would be considered a social aggregate.

Groups are studied at the **macro**- and **micro**-levels. Micro-level analysis involves the study of interpersonal relationships in groups and face-to-face interaction; while macro-level analysis involves the study of formal organizations and bureaucracies. At the micro-level, we define various types of groups on the basis of size and purpose. The smallest group is known as a *dyad*, a form identified by Simmel (1955), which refers to a group of two people. This is the building block of social relationships, and it is where we experience strong social bonds. For example, a married couple is considered a dyad. He further identified the *triad*, which he considered to be more stable in nature than the dyad. These 3-person groups are less fragile than dyads because a third person may relieve some of the pressure experienced by other group members.

Another important contribution of sociology was the identification of *primary* and *secondary* groups by Charles Horton Cooley (1864–1929). He characterized primary groups as those that were small/intimate, based largely on face-to-face interaction, and long-lasting. Some examples of primary groups are families or our closest friends. In contrast, secondary groups are characterized by large, impersonal groups and the relationships are typically not long-lasting. Examples of secondary groups include professional associations, academic clubs, and so on. Primary and secondary groups can also be differentiated by their goals and focus. Primary groups are often developed or created to meet emotional needs while secondary groups are often based around utilitarian purposes or to meet a goal. Thus, the way people within various groups feel about each other can be used as a way to determine what type they are.

Sociologists also distinguish between **in-** and **out-groups**. An **in-group** is a group toward which we feel loyalty and respect, and is similar to the definition of a primary group developed by Cooley. These are the people we associate with, think well of, and consider ourselves a part of ("us"). Alternately, **out-groups** are those we distance ourselves from and feel antagonism and contempt toward ("them"). We often compare ourselves against members of out-groups and view their behaviors and attitudes negatively. From a sociological standpoint this is important since it reinforces social solidarity by allowing us to identify an "us" versus "them" distinction. This helps to set up group boundaries and reinforce social norms (Ritzer and

Ryan 2010). Following this distinction, we are better able to understand what is referred to as **attribution error**. This occurs when we perceive members of out-groups in a negative way, regardless what the reality may be. Group identities are commonly organized on gender, race/ethnicity, class, and so on. A great example for understanding attribution error is to consider the following scenario (recognizing that we all make assumptions about people based on whether we perceive them as part of the in-group, "us," or the out-group, "them"). Let's say that you notice someone who you consider an *in-group* member carrying a weapon. Because they are an in-group member, you might assume that they must carry that weapon for protection. On the other hand, let's say you notice someone who is an *out-group* member carrying a weapon. In that case, you might assume that the person is carrying the weapon because they are hostile or violent. In either case, you've made an attribution error by assuming the reasons for carrying a weapon must be justified because, "they're one of us" in the case of the in-group member; or they're violent in the case of the out-group member. A sociologist would be quick to point out that many of the police shootings of young, unarmed black men may be better understood by considering how commonly we commit attribution errors on the basis of group membership.

Another type of group sociologists consider is the **reference group**. These are groups that you identify with, and you use as a standard for evaluating your own values, attitudes, and behaviors. These can also be thought of as our role models, and are commonly, but not always in-groups. Accordingly, in some cases, these groups may have positive or negative impacts. For example, students in the health sciences may aspire to be like the professional doctors and nurses they observe, and this serves as an important tool for professionalization (i.e. secondary socialization). Similarly, young children may look up to sports stars, which again has positive effects for the most part given that participation in sports results in an array of positive impacts. But, the effects may also be negative if these role models regularly engage in undesirable behavior, such as using performance enhancing drugs.

A great study that shows well how we attribute certain characteristics to entire groups of people (based on stereotypes we attach to reference groups as well and in- and out-groups) is shown in Fig. 4.2. Here, the stereotype content model (SCM) illustrates how a sample of students attributed positive characteristics to entire classes of people that make up the "in-group" from a larger societal standpoint (Cuddy et al. 2009). Accordingly, societal prototype groups (those that represent the mainstream values of society), or reference groups, and in-groups are identified as having positive characteristics. In opposite fashion those in out-groups, societally-speaking, are attributed worse characteristics.

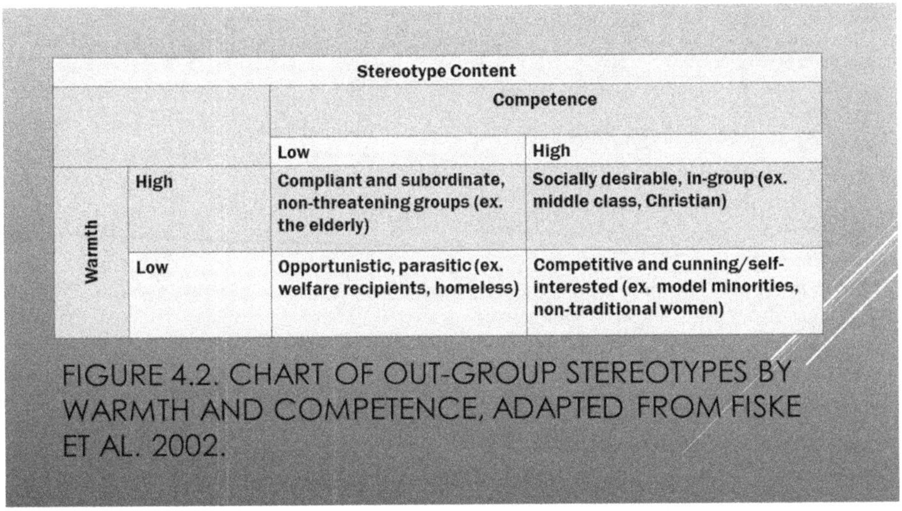

Stereotype Content			
		Competence	
		Low	High
Warmth	High	Compliant and subordinate, non-threatening groups (ex. the elderly)	Socially desirable, in-group (ex. middle class, Christian)
	Low	Opportunistic, parasitic (ex. welfare recipients, homeless)	Competitive and cunning/self-interested (ex. model minorities, non-traditional women)

FIGURE 4.2. CHART OF OUT-GROUP STEREOTYPES BY WARMTH AND COMPETENCE, ADAPTED FROM FISKE ET AL. 2002.

Fig. 4.2 Chart of out-group stereotypes by warmth and competence (Adapted from Fiske et al. 2002)

Fig. 4.3 Asch experiment (1958)

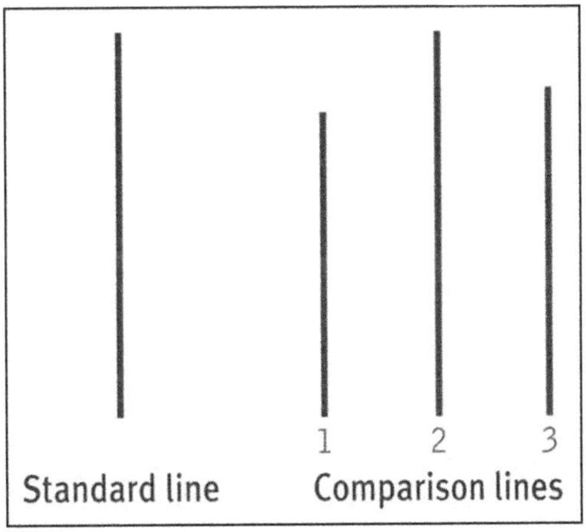

4.3.2 Conformity and Obedience

Another important aspect of groups has to do with conformity at the micro-level (and obedience to authority at the macro-level). Some of the most famous experiments in the social sciences came from our desire to understand how and why people behave differently in group setting and/or comply with orders of those in authority, even when those orders required irrational or unethical behaviors.

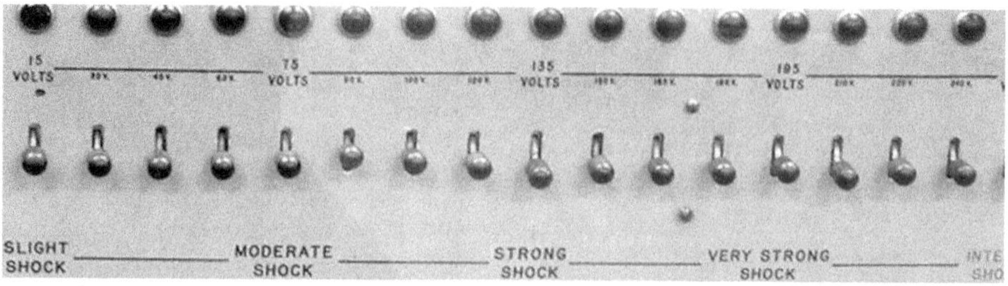

Fig. 4.4 Electric shock panel used in milgram study (Source: http://www.gina-perry.com/behind-the-shock/milgrams-obedience-experiments/)

In a groundbreaking study of conformity conducted by Solomon Asch (1907–1996), college students were asked to participate in a study on visual perception, in which they were asked to match the length of a line to three others (see Fig. 4.3). Unknown to the research subjects, a series people who were in on the experiment intentionally gave the wrong answer in front of the subjects. Surprisingly, the study revealed that one-third of the subjects consequently gave the wrong answer in order to conform. This research paved the way for later experiments that continued to show the importance of conformity.

In a study by Stanley Milgram (1933–1984), researchers sought to answer whether subjects would conform to/obey an authority even if it meant causing harm to another person. His research was borne out of a need to try and explain why the atrocities of the Holocaust happened, and was based on the notion that people will submit to legitimate authority created by bureaucracies (described in a later section). He recruited subjects to participate in a study on the effect of punishment on memory. The subjects were asked to take on the role of the "teacher" who would read a series of word pairs to the "learner". The "teachers" were asked to administer a shock to the learners who got responses incorrect. These shocks ranged from very minor to lethal (Fig. 4.4), and subjects were asked to increase the voltage with each additional wrong answer. What the subjects didn't know was that the "learners' were actually actors who were in on the experiment. As the voltage increased, the "learners" would increase the intensity of their complaints and finally stopped responding completely. The "teachers" became distressed over the decision to continue with the shocks, at which point the experimenter would read a script encouraging them to continue with the shocks. Shockingly, a majority of the subjects (65%) went all the way up to the highest voltage (which would've been deadly had the experiment been real). This experiment is especially important because it showed how most people will submit to a legitimate authority figure, i.e. a person in a lab coat, in this case, even if they have doubts about doing it. For actual footage of the experiment, visit: https://www.youtube.com/watch?v=PJFzqfLMBIw.

A final well-known experiment, that was recently made into a feature film was the Stanford Prison Experiment, was conducted by Philip Zimbardo in 1971. In this experiment, the researcher recruited male students at Stanford University to participate in a mock prison experiment. These men were screened to ensure they were well-adjusted, and then randomly assigned to act as guards or prisoners. To the surprise of the researcher, the students fully took on the roles they were assigned. In the case of the guards, they engaged in sadistic and abusive behaviors; while the prisoners did not question the authority of the guards and suffered extreme emotional disturbances. The experiment had to be cut short given the intensity of the ethics violations. It is used as an example of the importance of maintaining ethical standards in studies involving human subjects as well as one that illustrates the way specific group contexts can prompt extreme and unexpected behaviors (for more information see the resource links).

Generally, these studies illustrate the importance of *conformity*, and we should certainly recognize that some level of conformity is essential to maintaining groups. But, the studies also revealed that most people are susceptible to coercion, don't question authority, and will engage in unexpected and potentially harmful ways as a result. A related concept, developed to explain why people make poor decisions as part of a group, is called groupthink (Janis 1971). This describes the tendency for group members to engage in defective decision-making. **Groupthink** is characterized by high cohesion of the group, belief in the correctness of the group, negative stereotypes of the out-group, and rationalization of the behavior. Examples of groupthink include the torture of prisoners at Abu Ghraib, The Watergate Scandal, and the attack on Pearl Harbor.

4.4 Macro-Level (Formal Organizations)

At the macro-level, we study the structure of organizations and societies. As the process of industrialization continued into the modern era, society became increasingly rationalized. What is meant by this is that the personal relationships, customs, and practices dominant in traditional societies became replaced with rules and procedures set forth to maximize efficiency in modern societies. Traditional societies are characterized by personal relationships and obligation to others, while modern ones are based on rationality and organized around routine practices and centralization. Thus, **organizations** are complex, secondary groups with an identifiable membership that are developed to accomplish specific tasks or goals. They tend to be **formal organizations**, which are those that rationally designed, with explicit rules and procedures to meet their objectives. Today's society is characterized by the dominance of major organizations like our government, the NFL, major universities, Nike, and so on. Organizations can be further separated into different types on the basis of their purpose.

Max Weber focused on the study of **bureaucracies**, a specific type of formal organization, designed to maximize efficiency. The ideal type bureaucracy is characterized by: (1) laws or rules that govern participants and provide officials with the authority to enforce rules and regulations, (2) hierarchical arrangements of individuals within the organization, and (3) individuals perform functions/duties in accordance with their qualifications (Weber 1946). He further argued that this was the best way to meet the needs of a large, complex society.

The McDonaldization of society is a final concept developed by George Ritzer to understand the processes that characterize modern society. Formally, it refers to the process by which the principles of the fast-food restaurant are coming to dominate

In the Health Setting: Those who study health and health disparities have long studies the impacts of individual, or micro-level, impacts on health. Accordingly, these types of studies consider things like how interactions between physicians and patients may differ on the basis of class or race; or, how treatment recommendations may vary for some groups compared to others. Increasingly, researchers are also starting to examine the role of system-level (macro-) factors. In the book, *Unequal Treatment*, the influence of organizations on health outcomes is identified as a key priority. System-level factors include such things as the availability of healthcare services in an area, the way reimbursement procedures work, and the use of managed care systems. These things may produce barriers to care in underserved communities, and it is necessary to consider how they might produce disparities in treatment and care.

more spheres of society, in the U.S. and the world (Ritzer 2006). The five principles of McDonaldization include: efficiency, calculability, predictability, control, and the irrationality of rationality. Efficiency refers to the optimal process for completing tasks, as in an assembly line to prepare fast food very quickly. Calculability refers to an emphasis on costs and quantifying the process. Predictability refers to the consistency observed from one location to another. Control refers to the substitution of non-human for human technology (like a soda machine that automatically measures the ratio of syrup to soda water). Finally, irrationality of rationality highlights the negative consequences of this type of system. For example, many have linked fast food consumption to a widespread obesity epidemic. Certainly, it is easy to recognize the prevalence of this type of model in modern society, as it has come to characterize more than just fast food establishments. We can see evidence of this type of model present in various businesses including childcare and healthcare, among others.

Key Terms and Definitions

- **Social Interaction**: a social exchange between two or more individuals that is given meaning
  - **Verbal and Non-verbal Communication**: symbols used in social exchanges, e.g. a smile sends a message that others understand and interpret to mean friendliness
  - **Patient-provider Interaction**: exchange of information between doctor and patients that involves instrumental communication (information exchange focused on achievement of goals), and affective communication (the expression of feelings and emotions)

- **Social Support** (Content Category 8C): resources available from family, friends, and others in social networks; a factor that may prevent or act as a buffer against negative events
- **Social Isolation**: voluntary and involuntary lack of contact with others

- **Elements of Social Interaction**
  - **Status** (Content Category 8C): the social identity a person has, i.e. doctor, lawyer, woman, etc.
  - **Social Roles** (Content Category 8C): socially defined expectations that a person in a given social position follows
- **Socialization** (Content Category 7B): the development of the skills and competencies necessary for participation in society; involves the transmission of cultural patterns and norms of behavior occurring at the individual, organizational, and societal level.
  - **Nature vs. Nurture**: the debate over whether biological drives and impulses are more important or influential than social and environmental ones on human behavior and the development of self
  - **Social Construction of Gender**: refers to the idea that gender roles are a social construct that do not reflect true biological differences
  - **Doing Gender**: we act in accordance with gender roles as well as perceive others' behaviors in line with the expectations we have learned about gender roles
  - **Primary Socialization**: the earliest phase of socialization (infancy and childhood) in which we learn basic social skills and internalize norms and values. The family, peer groups, and schools are important agents in the primary socialization process.
  - **Secondary Socialization**: a phase of socialization that occurs throughout the life-course, it is often acquired by choice as one prepares for new stages in life
- **Agents of Socialization** (Content Category 7B): people and institutions that serve to communicate social facts; they act as key sources for the transmission of norms, values, and attitudes
  - The agents of socialization that sociologists consider to be main influences include: the family, schools, peers, religious organizations, the mass media, organized sports, and the workplace
- **Impression Management/Dramaturgical Approach** (Content Category 8C): a perspective developed by Erving Goffman; based on the idea that social actions are guided by performances. Using theater as a metaphor, individuals are social actors who actively manipulate the impressions perceived by others via perfor-

mances. The process is ever-evolving and dependent on the reactions of others. Thus, actors work to alter impressions as needed.

- **Groups** (Content Category 8C): collection of individuals who interact with one another, share goals and norms, and have a shared sense of belonging.
  - **Macro-level**: style of analysis which seeks to understand and explain large-scale social systems such as formal organizations and bureaucracy
  - **Micro-level**: Micro-level analysis involves the study of interpersonal relationships in groups and face-to-face interaction.
  - **In-group**: a group toward which we feel loyalty and respect; people we associate with, think well of, and consider ourselves a part of ("us")
  - **Out-group**: those we distance ourselves from and feel antagonism and contempt toward ("them"); we often compare ourselves against members of out-groups and view their behaviors and attitudes negatively
  - **Attribution Error**: when people perceive members of out-groups in a negative way, regardless what the reality may be
  - **Reference Group**: a group composed of members who serve as role models for others (who may or may not belong) and set the norms or standards of behavior
- **Social Networks** (Content Category 8C)
- **Formal Organizations**: complex, secondary groups with an identifiable membership; rationally designed, with explicit rules and procedures to meet their objectives.
  - **Bureaucracy**: the rule of officials; describes the way administration, execution, and enforcement of rules is socially organized
- **Conformity and Obedience to Authority** (Content Category 7B)
  - **Conformity**: the tendency of individuals to comply with or agree to various activities to reflect agreement with the group
  - **Obedience to Authority**: the tendency of individuals to submit to the demands of a person/entity perceived to have some legitimate authority; a concept used to explain the irrational or unexpected behaviors of individuals
    - Famous experiments: Studies including the Asch Conformity Study, Milgram Obedience Studies, and Stanford Prison Experiment all illustrate the power of group processes in altering individual behavior. They further show the importance of conformity to the group and in the case of the latter two, obedience to authority.
  - **Groupthink**: conformity to group values and ethics to the extent that members engage in defective decision-making

Activities and Research Examples

Activity 1: Online Interaction.

What are the benefits to online interaction? What are the disadvantages? Also, consider the increasing use of alternate forms of patient-provider interaction (tele-health, smart phone apps, video conferencing, etc.). How can these be used to improve accessibility for groups that experience barriers to accessing health? What are the potential problems with using such forms?

Activity 2: McDonadization.

Come up with an example of McDonaldization in a health setting. Do you see evidence of the characteristics' identified by Ritzer? Is this a positive or negative development? Does this contribute to health disparities?

Research Example 1: The Social Construction of Gender. The assignment of gender to infants who are intersexed offers an opportunity to think in a much more in-depth way about the social aspects of sex roles. Read the following article and engage in an in-class discussion about the factors that are considered and their inherently social nature. Article: Suzanne J. Kessler. 1990. "The Medical Construction of Gender: Case Management of Intersexed Infants," *Signs: Journal of Women in Culture and Society* 16(1): 3–26.

Resources, Links, and Recommended Readings

Help-Seeking and Health Behavior Recommended Readings:

Pescosolido, Bernice A. 1992. "Beyond Rational Choice: The Social Dynamics of How People Seek Help." *American Journal of Sociology*, 92(4): 1096–1138.
Andersen, R.M., 1995. Revisiting the Behavioral Model and Access to Medical Care: Does it Matter? *Journal of Health and Social Behavior* 36(1): 1–10.

Intersectionality Recommended Reading:

Crenshaw, Kimberlé. 1989. Demarginalizing the Intersection of Race and Sex: A Black Feminist Critique of Antidiscrimination Doctrine. *University of Chicago Legal Forum*, 1989: 139–168.
Collins, Patricia Hill. 1990. *Black Feminist Thought*. Cambridge: XX.

Patient Provider Interactions Recommended Readings:

Hibbard, Judith H., and Jessica Greene. 2013. "What the Evidence Shows about Patient Activation: Better Health Outcomes and Care Experiences; Fewer Data on Costs." *Health Affairs* 32(2): 207–214.
Haskard Zolnierek, K. B., & DiMatteo, M. R. 2009. "Physician Communication and Patient Adherence to Treatment: A Meta-analysis," *Medical Care*, 47(8): 826–834.
Institute of Medicine (US) Committee on Understanding and Eliminating Racial and Ethnic Disparities in Health Care; Smedley BD, Stith AY, Nelson AR, editors. *Unequal Treatment: Confronting Racial and Ethnic Disparities in Health Care*. Washington (DC): National Academies Press (US); 2003. Patient-Provider Communication: The Effect of Race and Ethnicity on Process and Outcomes of Healthcare. Available from: https://www.ncbi.nlm.nih.gov/books/NBK220354/

Caring with Compassion: A resource for students, medical providers, and educators that focuses on the knowledge and skilles needed to serve at-risk populations.

The website includes a curriculum that introduces the bio-psychosocial model for the provision of personalized care for at-risk patients. https://caringwithcompassion.org/resources/reference-guides

Human Rights Campaign: The Human Rights Campaign is America's largest civil rights organization working to achieve gay, lesbian, bisexual and transgender equality. By inspiring and engaging all Americans, HRC strives to end discrimination against GLBT citizens and realize a nation that achieves fundamental fairness and equality for all (http://www.hrc.org//).

McDonaldization Interview Series and Blog Postings on globalization, McDonaldization, and Consumption (George Ritzer): www.georgeritzer.com

Secret of the Wild Child (NOVA Documentary): A documentary that explores the experiences of a child who remained largely socially isolated in her developmental years. (http://www.pbs.org/wgbh/nova/education/programs/2112_wildchil.html)

The Stanford Prison Experiment: The official Stanford Prison Experiment website features extensive information about the classic psychology experiment including background on recruitment, discussion questions, and an extensive series of links to additional resources. (www.prisonexp.org)

U.C. Berkeley, Centers for Educational Justice and Community Engagement, LGBTQ+ Definition of Terms: http://ejce.berkeley.edu/geneq/resources/lgbtq-resources/definition-terms

Study Questions

1. Define social norms and give an example of how they may vary by context or from one group to another.

***Example Exam Question:** "Although socio-cultural patterns of drinking vary, excessive alcohol consumption is most accurately described as:

A. an excuse for social loafing.
B. an example of deviant behavior.
C. a medium for social facilitation.
D. a sign of peer pressure." (AAMC 2012: 117).

*For more information, visit https://students-residents.aamc.org/applying-medical-school/article/whats-mcat-exam/ for more information

References

AHRQ Toolkit Helps Health Care Organizations and Providers Communicate With Patients and Families When Harm Occurs. (2016). Content last reviewed May 2016. Rockville: Agency for Healthcare Research and Quality. http://www.ahrq.gov/news/newsroom/press-releases/2016/candor.html

Anyon, J. (1980). Social class and the hidden curriculum of work. *Journal of Education, 1*, 67–92.

Appelrouth, S. A., & Edles, L. D. (2012). *Classical and contemporary sociological theory* (2nd ed.). Los Angeles: Sage Press.

Association of American Medical Colleges (AAMC). (2012). *Preview guide for the MCAT 2015 exam* (2nd ed.). www.aamc.org/MCAT2015
Association of American Medical Colleges (AAMC). (2015). *The official guide to the MCAT exam (MCAT2015)* (4th ed.). Washington, DC: The Association of American Medical Colleges.
Berkman, L. F. (2000). Social support, social networks, social cohesion and health. *Social Work in Health Care, 31*(2), 3–14. doi:10.1300/J010v31n02_02.
Butler, J. (1991). *Gender trouble: Feminism and the subversion of identity*. New York: Routledge.
Connell, R. (1987, 2014). *Gender and power; society, the person, and sexual politics*. CA: Stanford University Press.
Cuddy, A. J. C., Fiske, S. T., Kwan, V. S. Y., Glick, P., Demoulin, S., Leyens, J.-P., & Ziegler, R. (2009). Stereotype content model across cultures: Towards universal similarities and some differences. *The British Journal of Social Psychology/The British Psychological Society, 48*(0 1), 1–33.
Dovidio, J. F., Penner, L. A., Albrecht, T. L., Norton, W. E., Gaertner, S. L., & Shelton, J. N. (2008). Disparities and distrust: The implications of psychological processes for understanding racial disparities in health and health care. *Social Science & Medicine, 67*(3), 478–486.
Fiske, S. T., Cuddy, A. J. C., Glick, P., & Xu, J. (2002). A model of (often mixed) stereotype content: Competence and warmth respectively follow from perceived status and competition. *Journal of Personality and Social Psychology, 82*(6), 878–902.
Galdas, P. M., Cheater, F., & Marshall, P. (2005). Men and health help-seeking behaviour: Literature review. *Journal of Advanced Nursing, 49*(6), 616–623.
Granovetter, M. S. (1973). The strength of weak ties. *American Journal of Sociology, 78*(6), 1360–1380.
Goffman, E. (1959). *The presentation of self in everyday life*. New York: Doubleday Anchor Books.
Guo, G. (2005). Twin studies: What canthey tell us about nature and nurture. *Contexts, 4*(3), 43–47.
Hampton, K. N., Sessions, L. F., & Her, E. J. (2011). Core networks, social isolation, and new media: How internet and mobile phone use is related to network size and diversity. *Information Communication and Society, 14*(1), 130–155.
Haskard Zolnierek, K. B., & DiMatteo, M. R. (2009). Physician communication and patient adherence to treatment: A meta-analysis. *Medical Care, 47*(8), 826–834.
House, J. S., Landis, K. R., & Umberson, D. (1988). Social relationships and health. *Science, 241*, 540–545.
Janis, I. L. (1971). Groupthink. *Psychology Today*, 5(6), 43–46.
McPherson, M., Smith-Lovin, L., & Brashears, M. E. (2006). Social isolation in America: Changes in core discussion networks over two decades. *American Sociological Review, 71*(3), 353–375.
PEW Research Center. (2016). *Three Technology Revolutions*. http://www.pewinternet.org/three-technology-revolutions/ Accessed 27 June 2016.
Ritzer, G. (2006). Globalization and McDonaldization: Does it all amount to… nothing. *Mcdonaldization: The Reader*. Pine Forge Press.
Ritzer, G., & Michael Ryan, J. (Eds.). (2010). *The concise encyclopedia of sociology*. Oxford: Wiley.
Smith, K. P., & Christakis, N. A. (2008). Social networks and health. *Annual Review of Sociology, 34*, 405–429.
Spitz, R. A. (1945). Hospitalism: An inquiry into the genesis of psychiatric conditions in early childhood. *Psychoanalytic Study of the Child, 1*, 53–74.
Stewart, M., Brown, J. B., Donner, A., McWhinney, I. R., Oates, J., Weston, W. W., et al. (2000). The impact of patient-centered care on outcomes. *Journal of Family Practice, 49*, 796–804.
Thoits, P. (1995). Stress, coping, and social support processes: Where are we? what next? *Journal of Health and Social Behavior, 36*(Suppl. 1), 53–79.
Umberson, D., & Montez, J. K. (2010). Social relationships and health a flashpoint for health policy. *Journal of Health and Social Behavior, 51*(1 suppl), S54–S66.
Weber, M. 1946. Bureaucracy/From Max Weber. *Essays in Sociology* (trans. and ed. H. H. Gerth, & C. W. Mills). London: Oxford University Press.
Weitzman, L. J., Eifler, D., Hokada, E., & Ross, C. (1972). Sex-Role socialization in picture books for preschool children. *American Journal of Sociology, 77*(6), 1125–1150.
West, C., & Zimmerman, D. H. (1987). Doing gender. *Gender and Society, 1*(2), 125–151. http://www.jstor.org/stable/189945.

Chapter 5
Culture

Objectives

- Introduce and define culture and related concepts
- Understand how cultural norms affect human behavior (Content Category 7B)
- Understand how ethnocentrism and cultural relativism affect the way we think about others (Content Category 8B)
- Understand how culture shapes our experiences and interactions with others (Content Category 9A)

Foundational Concepts 7, 8 & 9

Concept 7

"Biological, psychological, and sociocultural factors influence behavior and behavior change...

Category 7B focuses on how social factors, such as groups and social norms, affect behavior." (AAMC 2015: 245).

In particular we answer the question: How do social norm, sanctions, folkways, mores, and taboos affect our behavior?

Clinical Example: "To truly understand and address the health consequences of smoking, contemporary physicians use biomedical knowledge of gas exchange, oxidative stress…To best serve their patients, they also need to understand why patients choose to smoke and how to facilitate behavioral change through building intrinsic motivation" (AAMC 2011: 14).

Concept 8

"Psychological, sociocultural, and biological factors influence the way we think about ourselves and others, as well as how we interact with others...

(continued)

G. Garcia-Alexander et al., *Social Foundations of Behavior for the Health Sciences*,
DOI 10.1007/978-3-319-64950-4_5

Category 8B focuses on the attitudes and beliefs that influence social interaction." (AAMC 2015 pg. 250) Herein, we will consider and describe the ways in which ethnocentrism and cultural relativism affect our attitudes about and our behavior toward others.

Concept 9

"Cultural and social differences influence well-being...

Category 9A focuses on the link between social structures and human interactions." (AAMC 2015 Pg. 255) Culture should be understood as a core component of the social structure. In this chapter, we will define the elements of culture and describe the ways in which culture influences patients' perceptions of health and disease, the health care team, and therapeutic interventions.

5.1 What Is Culture?

Culture is a very broad term that encompasses nearly every aspect of our day-to-day lives. It includes our values and rules that govern our behavior, our language, the way we dress, our tools and technology, music, art, and religion. Our beliefs about health and health care are also part of our culture. Throughout this chapter we'll learn about the importance of culture in shaping our lives and how it may lead to differences in expectations, understanding, treatment adherence, and perceptions related to patient-physician interactions. Having a good understanding of culture, especially where health beliefs are concerned are particularly important for health care providers, who must understand their patients' values and beliefs in order to provide culturally appropriate care.

Culture includes both **material culture,** the physical objects, tools, art, and clothing; as well as **symbolic, or non-material culture** such as beliefs, values, and norms. Much of our knowledge about human cultures comes from the study of anthropology, which uses in-depth description (ethnography) to help us understand the differences between societies. As sociologists, we focus on how culture allows us to engage in meaning-making and can be loosely thought of our way of life.

Material and non-material culture are inextricably linked. Consider, for example the activity tracker. In contemporary western societies activity trackers have become commonplace. About 50% of Americans currently own an activity tracker. Most of the remaining half likely knows what they are. In fact 57% of Americans responding to a recent survey indicated they had plans to purchase an activity tracker in the next year. (PwC 2016) This increasingly ubiquitous technology – an example of material culture – is also a reflection of our values, or non-material culture. The U.S. is an extremely health conscious culture. Most people that own trackers do so because of the perceived health benefits. Would the activity tracker be as wildly popular in a society that cares less about health and exercise than the U.S.? (Fig. 5.1)

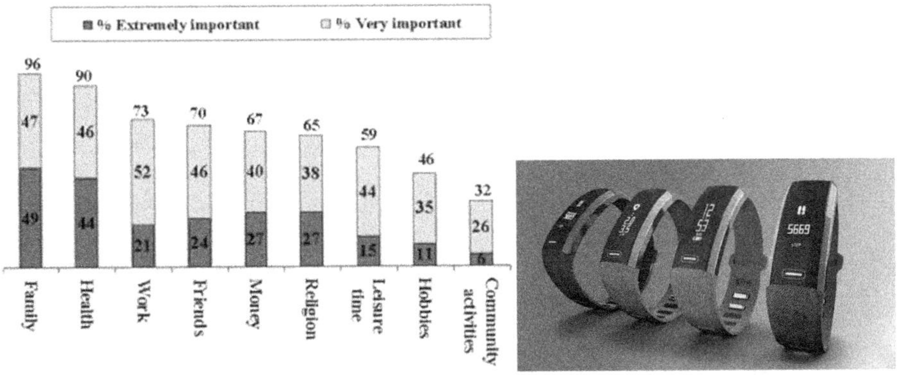

Fig. 5.1 American values (Source: Moore, David W. 2003. Family, health, most important aspects of life. Gallup Poll. http://www.gallup.com/poll/7504/family-health-most-important-aspects-life.aspx, CCO public domain)

5.2 Values, Beliefs and Norms

Values, beliefs and social norms are all part of culture. **Values** are abstract ideas about what is desirable or not desirable, right or wrong, good or bad. Values also form the glue of society, a shared sense of values is fundamental to social cohesion. One of the most common ways Sociologists understand shared values in a society is by asking a large number of people about what is important to them. In a poll of Americans, for example, most people will say they value their families, heath, and their work. A **belief** is simply an idea about what is true. For example, most Americans now believe that humans are affecting climate change, and that smoking is bad for your health. As with values, sociologists often try to understand similarities and difference in beliefs in order to better understand human behavior and differences between societies. Values and beliefs form the basis for **social norms**, which are unspoken rules that guide our day-to-day behavior. Values, beliefs and norms often interact in complicated ways. Consider smoking – rates of smoking have been declining rapidly over the past several decades, and continue to decline (see Fig. 5.2). In the 1950s, when about half of Americans were smokers, social norms surrounding smoking were very different. It was common for people to smoke cigarettes at work, inside their homes, and at social gatherings. Smoking was, in fact, a social norm. Today, this seems rather strange. Rates of smoking have been steadily declining since the 1950s, reflecting changes in the evidence and attitudes about the health implications of smoking. Smoking, in fact, is no longer a social norm. But smoking laws were slow to follow changes in norms. It wasn't until 1988, when only about 1/3 of American's still smoked cigarettes that smoking laws were initiated on airplanes in the US, and not until 2000, that smoking was banned on all airlines. (USDHHS 2017).

In the case of smoking, it's clear that behavior began to change long before laws were enacted that influenced smoking behavior. That is, social norms changed, and

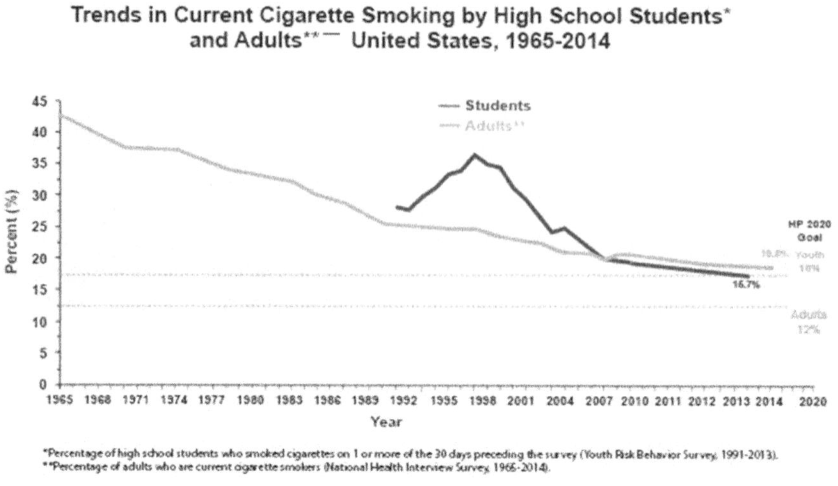

Fig. 5.2 Trends in Cigarette smoking in the United States 1965–2014 (Source: *CDC* http://www.cdc.gov/tobacco/data_statistics/tables/trends/cig_smoking/index.htm)

smoking became less prevalent long before laws were enacted. However, it's also clear that changes in laws have also continued to change behavior. Workplace bans on smoking, for example, are credited with further reducing declining smoking rates in the US. (Evans et al. 1999) Nevertheless, in the case of social norms relating to smoking, it is clear that what's considered normative, or socially acceptable, has changed over time and the once commonplace cigarette is now relatively rare.

Norms are enforced, sometimes subtly, sometimes not-so-subtly through **sanctions**, both positive (**rewards**) and negative (punishment). Consider what would happen if someone lit a cigarette in a social gathering where no one else was smoking. How would others react? In most cases, the people around them would simply move away – shunning is a type of sanction and in fact can be a relatively powerful sanction. However, it's also very possible, even likely, that the smoker would be chastised or harassed. Some norms are considerably less serious and related to social etiquette – what is considered polite. These norms are referred to as **Folkways**, and usually carry very light, if any real sanctions. **Mores** refer to social norms that most would consider to be more serious, and have a moral component to them. Although this is changing, having a baby out of wedlock would be considered an example of a more. Sanctions for mores are more serious than for folkways. A **taboo,** is a behavior that violates a social norm that carries a strong moral component. In many cultures, taboos are expressed in laws with significant punishments. Though there are few universal taboos, killing someone is a taboo in nearly all cultures.

5.3 Language and Symbols

Language, simply put, is a system of symbols that allows humans to communicate with each other. Language allows us to record our past, and transmit information about objects and ideas into the future. As such, it is the essential tool for cultural transmission, the passing down of culture from one generation to the next. According to linguists Edward Sapir and Benjamin Lee Whorf, language actually influences how we think and behave. Their *Sapir-Whorf hypothesis*, often referred to as the linguistic relatively hypothesis, suggests that our very thoughts are constrained by the language we learn. Compared to English speakers, who speak about time as discrete units (seconds, hours, minutes) and have phrases like "save time" or "spend time" the Hopi Indians have no such language, and as a consequence have a very different view of time. Similarly, the famous example of Eskimos having many more words for snow than other cultures suggests that because snow is so much more important to Native Alaskan Inuits, they have a number of different words to describe snow and thus perceive snow differently than other cultures. However, the linguistic relatively hypothesis remains controversial because of lack of empirical support. That is, how can you really prove that one society thinks about snow differently in specific ways that are connected to the words they use to describe it?

Language certainly reflects both the values and norms of a culture. For example, extended family hierarchies are much more important in Chinese families than in American culture. And there are many more specific words used to describe family members in the Chinese language because it is important to know whom you are talking about. Unlike in the English language, where people refer to grandparents as simply grandma or grandpa, in Chinese, relatives all have more specific referents based on whether they are your mother's mother "wài pó" or your father's mother "zǔmǔ."

Because the meaning of language is inherently connected to culture, just knowing the words in a language does not allow someone to effectively communicate in that language. This is why language education emphasizes studying abroad, in order to enhance a student's understanding of the cultural meanings attached. In the U.S. for example, the word "sick" is often used to denote something that is "cool" and not physical illness. Imagine how easy it would be for a non-native speaker to misunderstand the phrase "that party was totally sick." Cultural context is very important.

In the Health Setting Language barriers not only make communication difficult, but they can be very dangerous in health care encounters. So much so that the federal government has required any medical care provider who receives federal funds (Medicare or Medicaid) to provide "linguistic access" to patients who have "limited English proficiency (LEP). This means that appropriate language services must be provided to all patients. Since then, many states require medical interpreters to be certified to ensure that language interpreters are able to interpret medical terms appropriately.

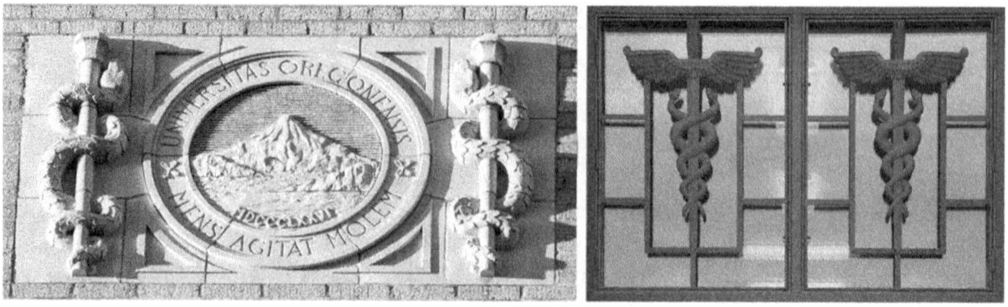

Fig. 5.3 The Caduceus and the Rod of Asclepius (*Left* – Source: McClintick, Daniel, "Multnomah Pavilion," OHSU Digital Commons, accessed September 7, 2017, https://www.ohsu.edu/custom/library/digital-collections/items/show/27031; (*Right* – "Baird Hall," OHSU Digital Commons, accessed September 7, 2017, https://www.ohsu.edu/custom/library/digital-collections/items/show/13919)

Symbols are objects or images that convey meaning, and often represent cultural beliefs. Their meanings often evoke powerful emotions. The meanings of symbols can vary over time, and from place to place. In medicine, for example, no symbol is better known than the caduceus, which is sometimes represented as a winged rod, with two snakes intertwined. The symbol however, is actually a misrepresentation. (Friedlander 1992) The caduceus comes from the Greek god Hermes, god of commerce, and is a symbol of business or trade rather than medical care. The ancient symbol of medical care is actually the Rod of Asclepius, which is a staff with no wings and one snake. This rod is associated with the Greek god of healing and medicine. In some cases, as on the front of a Medical School building (Fig. 5.3), the correct symbol, the Rod of Asclepius is used, but incorrectly referred to as a Caduceus. In other cases, such as the Army Medical Core, the symbol of Hermes is correctly identified as the Caduceus but used as a symbol for medical care, which is based on a misinterpretation. Nevertheless, these examples show that the origin of a symbol is not what gives it meaning. Even though most of us don't know the history of the caduceus, where it comes from or how the meaning has changed over time, both symbols are commonly referred as the caduceus, and both carry the same meaning in the contemporary US. The power of symbols lie in their associations. Another very clear example of a transformed symbol is the swastika, one of the most recognizable symbols in western culture. It was once a Buddhist symbol of peace and harmony and had nothing to do with racism or anti-Jewish sentiment. However, by virtue of its association with the Nazi party in Germany, it has been transformed into the universally recognized symbol it is today. The Swastika, for many people, conveys a powerful and negative emotional response, which is certainly not part of its original meaning.

5.4 Rituals

Rituals are group activities or actions, often performed at specific times and places that serve to unite individuals around culturally important values. Rituals often involve the use of symbols to reinforce a shared sense of meaning and purpose. In the US, for example, it's so common to celebrate birthdays with a birthday and candles, and by singing happy birthday and blowing out the candles that the image of a round cake with candles is virtually synonymous with "Happy Birthday." Religious rituals have long been studied by sociologists as a way of understanding the mechanisms through which social solidarity is maintained. In fact, one of the fathers of sociology, Emile Durkheim, examined how primitive societies used rituals as a way of strengthening and reinforcing the bonds between group members. However, rituals are not just religious. Sports involve a number of rituals as well. Consider that most sporting events involve singing a national anthem, displaying of national flags, and some sort of show of respect such as standing or removing hats. These rituals serve to reinforce emotional bonds between group members and emphasize the importance group membership.

A number of Native American tribes use traditional tobacco as part of their ceremonies. This ritual use of tobacco has a number of social and religious meanings. It is given as a gift, burned as part of a blessing, and smoked in social gatherings. There are a number of misconceptions about ritual use of traditional tobacco, which does not present the same health hazards as does the use of commercial tobacco. Traditional tobacco is grown and processed without the use of dangerous chemicals or additives, is not used by children, is not always inhaled, and is reserved for special occasions. Because traditional tobacco does not have added nicotine or other chemicals, and used only in ritual practice, it does not carry the same risk of addiction as does commercial tobacco. However, the large commercial tobacco industry has worked hard to promote their products to youth, and thus the rate of commercial tobacco use among Native American youth is relatively high. In order to curtail commercial tobacco use while keeping alive the sacred traditions associated with traditional tobacco use, there is a growing movement in public health to "keep it sacred" and emphasize the differences between the ritual use of traditional tobacco and use of commercial tobacco. For more information see the website: http://keepitsacred.itcmi.org/.

5.5 Cultural Lag and Culture Shock

As technology continues to increase at faster pace, there are numerous examples of how these changes have disrupted the fabric of our society. **Cultural lag** refers to the situation where social norms are disrupted by rapid social and technological change. An often cited, and very relevant example of cultural lag is how technological changes in fertility treatments and birth practices have created a need to redefine how we think about family. When a lesbian couple has a baby using donated sperm, how are we to understand the sperm donor's relationship to the child? Does it matter if the couple knows the donor? Does the donor have a right to a relationship with the child? There really are no right or wrong answers here, which can make modern family life rather difficult, as there are no norms, yet, associated with our new family arrangements.

In comparison, **Culture Shock** is the personal confusion and discomfort that is felt when being confronted with an unfamiliar culture. Culture shock is something that health care providers need to be aware of and sensitive to as our society grows increasingly diverse. As an example, most Muslims consider personal modesty to be a very important part of their culture. They have strict rules about gender segregation, and are used to having segregated medical facilities. (Rabin 2010) In American culture, we don't tend to segregate medical facilities, and it is not considered unusual or inappropriate for a physician to treat a patient of the opposite sex.

> *In the Health Setting:* Imagine how difficult it would be for a Muslim woman with strict beliefs to arrive in an emergency room and find herself alone in the room with a male doctor. To most American women, this would not be terribly concerning. To a Muslim woman, this could be a difficult and untenable situation.

5.6 Ethnocentrism and Cultural Relativism

In a progressively diverse society there are increased opportunities to interact with people from other cultures. In practice this is not always easy. There is a natural tendency for all of us to favor our own culture, and what is familiar to us. This tendency to look down on other cultures, and judge them using your own cultural standards is referred to as **Ethnocentrism**. Being ethnocentric means regarding other cultures as inferior to your own, and failing to take into account others' views about the importance of their own norms, values, and behaviors. Most people have this tendency to see their own culture as superior, in fact many social scientists believe that this tendency may have deep psychological and even evolutionary roots. However, whether this is nature or nurture, it is certainly something we can learn to understand and address in our behavior. Ethnocentrism can be harmful, especially in the healthcare context, and it's important to be aware of this tendency and guard against it. In the example above, failing to take into account the importance of modesty in Muslim culture means that health care providers would not be able to effectively treat female patients without taking into account their preferences for gender-segregated healthcare. The opposite of ethnocentrism is **cultural relativism** which means judging a society or culture by its own standards. This does not mean always agreeing with other cultures, but it does mean trying to understand and act on others' preferences (also see Chap. 6: Race and Ethnicity).

Working in a healthcare context requires practicing cultural relativity. Unlike mainstream American culture where health and illness are viewed primarily in biomedical terms, many other cultures including a number of Asian and Latin American cultures see health and illness in spiritual terms as well. For them illness is not simply caused by bacteria, viral infections, or the disease process. Many patients from diverse backgrounds believe that healing the body requires addressing the spirit and not simply using medical treatment. Practitioners of Western (allopathic) medicine have often been insensitive to the cultural views of diverse patients. This is one of the major causes of health disparities. When providers fail to acknowledge the unique values and beliefs of their patients, the resulting distrust leads to low rates of medical care use and failure to follow-through with treatment guidelines for treatable chronic diseases like diabetes and heart disease. Over the past several decades cultural competence has been improving though. One such example of this is that some hospitals are recruiting spiritual healers to work alongside medical care providers to attend to patients' desires for addressing spiritual needs of patients, which also effectively increases trust and the likelihood of better health outcomes.

Understanding, tolerance, and acting on patients' cultural preferences is an important part of providing high quality medical care. Cultural competence in healthcare has been found to improve health outcomes and patient satisfaction for racial and ethnic minorities. So much so, that providing cultural competence training is now a routine part of medical training. In fact, it's one of the major reasons that Sociology is now required on the medical college entrance exam, and why you are likely reading this book!

5.7 Assimilation and Multiculturalism

Assimilation, also commonly referred to in the public health literature as acculturation refers to adopting the cultural elements, the values, norms, language, dress and traditions of the dominant culture of the host country. Historically, this was viewed in relatively simple terms as a linear process in which subsequent generations of immigrant families came to use the language and adopt the norms and values of the host country until eventually their previous language and ways of life were completely replaced with those of the dominant American culture. In this way of thinking there are really only two states of being, immigrants either remained "backward" and unassimilated, or essentially "Americanized". This way of thinking about assimilation generally views the economic success of immigrant populations in terms of their own willingness to conform, to "get with the program" and choose to fit into their host country. The process of assimilation is not that simple of course. Rather than this "unidimensional" acculturation model, acculturation is understood today as being more "bidimensional." This means that immigrant groups tend to retain their own culture, and selectively adopt elements of American culture.

The extent to which various immigrant groups actually accept American cultural values and beliefs varies considerably. The ability of immigrant groups to become accepted into mainstream American culture and succeed financially, politically, and socially depends on a number of things that are outside of the control of immigrant groups. Some of those things include American views about immigrants in general, or views about immigrants from certain host countries. Another important factor that influences the acceptance of immigrants in the U.S. is race. As is discussed more fully in Chap. 6, race is considered a socially constructed category, which is largely based on skin color. Immigrant groups with lighter skin tone often do better economically. Light skinned European immigrants have an easier time gaining acceptance and succeeding economically that more recent immigrants from Asia or Latin America who must contend with racial discrimination (Hersch 2017). As the chart (Fig. 5.4) shows below, America, just like many European nations, remain deeply divided in their views of immigrants; although approximately half of Americans still indicate that they think immigrants make our country stronger.

From the perspective of immigrants, there are both positive and negative aspects of acculturation as well. The rapid growth of Latino populations in the US has led public health researchers to carefully study the impact of acculturation on the health of Latino immigrants. In general, compared with those who stay in their home countries, or who come to the US, but don't adopt the American lifestyle, Latino immigrants who assimilate into American culture are more like to visit the doctor, use preventive health care like cancer screening, and are more likely to exercise. In other words, there are a lot of positive effects of acculturation on health behavior. On the other hand, acculturation also leads to higher rates of drug and alcohol use, cigarette smoking, and diseases like diabetes, asthma, and hypertension. (LaVeist 2012) These health effects are due to a number of factors including changes in diet, as well as stress associated with "becoming a minority" in the U.S.

From its origins, America has been called a melting pot, a place where people of different ethnic backgrounds come together to create something new. The metaphor of the melting pot, however, suggests that diverse cultures melt together, assimilate into a single culture with the same language and values. By contrast, **multiculturalism** (also referred to as accommodation or the salad bowl model) means acknowledging, accepting, and celebrating diverse cultures equally. Despite being thought of as a melting pot, the United States in some ways exemplifies a multicultural society. There are a number of examples of this. One is the federal government's requirement that health care interpreters be provided to patients who don't speak English. The increased emphasis on cultural competence training for health providers is another. To some extent, given the increasing diversity of the United States, a certain amount of multiculturalism is inevitable. Forty percent of Americans are not white, and one-third of American's don't speak English in their home. This increased diversity provides the backdrop against which we must manage our educational system, our workplaces, and our communities.

Our divided political views about immigrants is quite instructive, however, and in many ways the United States remains conflicted about adopting multicultural practices and policies. As recently as 1998, voters in the state of California passed a law requiring English only education in the schools. In 2016, this law was repealed by an overwhelming majority of voters, paving the way for bilingual education in the state of California.

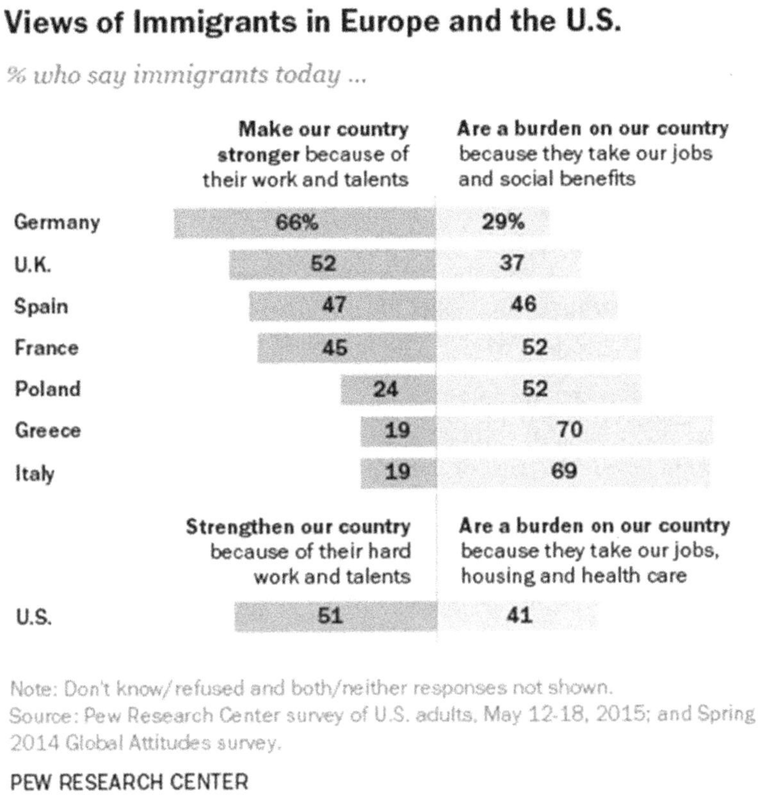

Fig. 5.4 Views of immigrants in Europe and the US (Source: http://www.pewresearch.org/fact-tank/2015/09/24/what-americans-europeans-think-of-immigrants/ft_09-24-15_europeimmigrants/)

5.8 Subcultures and Countercultures

Understanding concepts such as cultural relativism, assimilation, and multiculturalism all assume an understanding of what the "dominant culture" is. That is, to what cultural standards do we expect immigrants to assimilate? The definition of dominant cultures is simply the culture of the numerically, politically, or economically dominant group. This means that the values and norms of White, middle class, Christian, America form the cultural "standard" in the U.S. This explains the strong opposition by many to expand the officially recognized language to include Spanish. Similarly, the dominant cultural standard for the American family is still the married, heterosexual, two-parent nuclear family that lives together with their children in a single-family dwelling. Although this family type does not represent the majority of American families, it is, nonetheless, the yardstick used by some to judge others (see more on contemporary families in Chap. 7).

Of course, most of us don't fit neatly within the dominant culture. Most people are part of one or more groups, or **subcultures** that have unique norms, values, even language that sets them apart from mainstream society. Subcultures can include commonplace groups like surfers, skateboarders, and music-based subcultures (hip-hop, heavy metal, electronic dance music). Each of these groups have their own style of dress, language, and behavioral rules that would not be recognized outside the group. These subgroups however, are not particularly at odds with mainstream culture. They tend to focus on shared interest. When the shared interest, though, runs deeply opposed to mainstream or dominant culture then a subculture would be considered **counterculture.** As implied by the name, a counterculture is a special type of subculture whose norms, values and attitudes are in direct conflict or opposition to mainstream culture. The most commonly used example of a counterculture is the hippies of the 1960s and 70s. Timothy Leary's now famous charge to "tune in, turn on, drop out" exemplified the hippies who emphasized sexual freedom, drug use, and avoiding the daily grind of formal occupations. Of course, what represents "outside the mainstream" is subject to change. This point is made quite clearly by the rapid expansion of Tattoos in America. Only a few years ago, tattoos were a significant visible symbol of counterculture. Now, nearly one-third of all Americans have one or more tattoos, and nearly half of all Millennials do! (The Harris Poll 2016) (Poll 2016).

5.9 Mass Media and Popular Culture

Mass Media refers to all forms of mass communication designed to reach large anonymous audiences including newspapers, radio, television, streaming video, and internet sources such as websites, blogs, and social media. Because it's so pervasive, mass media exerts a tremendous influence on American culture. Today, Americans spend the majority of their waking hours taking in mass communication through screens on TVs, smartphones, tablets, and computers. Adults spend more than 8 h per day on screens (Nielsen Q1 report), mostly watching TV (5 h) and using the internet and social media (3 h). Youth, or those ages 8–18, also spend a great deal of time interacting with screens. Tweens (8–12 years) spend nearly 6 h per day on screens, mostly TV (2.5 h) and playing video games (1.3 h); while teenagers spend a whopping 9 h a day taking in media. Most of that time is spent on TV (2.6 h), listening to music (2 h), playing video games (1 h) and on social media (1 h).

Mass media is produced by a relatively small number of large corporations that exert tremendous control over the content. In fact a very small number of corporations own most of the television, radio, and print media content that we view. Time, Disney, News Corporation, Viacom, and Bertelsmann are among only a handful of corporations that effectively control much of the media. Both the content of mass media, and the products they sell through advertising make up **popular culture** – the mass-produced ideas, images, and entertainment designed to be accessible to a large audience.

Since people spend so much time taking in mass media it is important to understand how mass media affects our social norms. Does corporate media actually create popular culture and the values, attitudes, and ideas that form the basis of day-to-day social interaction? Or, do they simply act as a mirror, reflecting the cultural values and norms of society? While there are arguments for both, there is no denying that a small number companies control the media, and that popular culture is deeply intertwined with consumer culture – to the benefit of corporate advertisers. One of the clearest examples of strong ties between corporate media and popular culture is the ever-expanding industry of product placement. Product placement is when a character in a television show or movie uses a product as part of the show itself. Sponsors pay millions of dollars to have television and movie characters wear Nike shoes, drink Pepsi or eat Cheetos. Although this is nothing new, mass media companies are now going beyond product placement to make the products themselves part of the art. A company called Maven Strategies connects producers of alcohol, watches and other products with rap stars who receive advertising cash to include those products in their songs. When you hear rap musicians sing about their watch, their champagne, or their shoes, they are probably getting paid to do it. Most often as we watch our televisions, listen to our radios, or even surf the internet, we understand that commercials are trying to sell us products. But, we don't usually stop and reflect on how the television shows, movies, and even the songs we listen to are also trying to convince us to purchase a product.

The reach of the media not only exerts a powerful influence on our consumer culture, but Noam Chomsky argues that the production of news by a small number of corporate elites exerts a strong influence on both the content and the views expressed in journalism and television news. Both by choosing what to report, and importantly what not to report, the news media tells us what is important, and can influence public perception to serve the needs of wealthy elites. This view suggests that mainstream media is little more than corporate and government propaganda designed to sway a passive viewing audience. In their book Manufacturing Consent, Herman and Chomsky (1988) identify a number of specific processes through which this occurs. First, corporate control of the media means that views that contradict or challenge the corporations or their advertisers will be suppressed. Second, the media themselves rely on the government officials and corporate leaders to act as sources in news stories about important events. Therefore viewers get only the "official story." Finally, the media serves to focus our attention on a common enemy as a way of generating passive support for furthering policies that serve the elites. During the cold war, news stories focused on Russia as an enemy. Now, Chomsky argues, we are doing the same with the War on Terror. Since virtually all mainstream media is run as a for-profit enterprise that is funded by advertisers, we should be asking ourselves how much control these companies have on what is reported and who profits.

Another important area of mass media influence is the promotion of racial and gender *stereotypes*. Television and movies, in particular, continue to promote racial and ethnic stereotypes in a number of ways. First, ethnic characters are most often portrayed in stereotyped roles. African Americans and other minority groups are very often absent from television and movies, and when they are included they are portrayed as gangsters and criminals. This serves to reinforce racial stereotypes. This process is similar to news media, which selectively reports crimes committed by minorities. As an example, a study of crime reporting in California compared news reports with official crime statistics (Dixon and Linz 2000). These authors found that Black criminals made up 37% of the news stories and Whites only 21%. If you watch the news you would think that Blacks commit almost twice as many crimes as Whites. However in reality, Blacks made up only 21% of those arrested and Whites made up 28%. This study illustrates how the media are more likely to report on crimes committed by minorities, and less likely to report on crimes by Whites, which reinforces negative stereotypes about minorities.

Gender stereotypes are also commonplace in mass media. Despite decades of recognition and widespread criticism, images of women in virtually every media space from billboards, to print media to television and movies continue to emphasize extreme thinness and unnatural proportions augmented by surgery and digitally enhanced photos. In fact, the main change in the twenty-first century isn't the prevalence of extreme images, it's the increased ability of technology to digitally enhance them. The prevalence of ideal-type images continue to exert a negative influence on young women who compare themselves to the impossible standards of beauty. The constant exposure to idealized images has been shown to promote negative body image and eating disorders. (Cohen and Blaszczynski 2015) This trend continues to expand into social media. Recent studies of Facebook show that photos posted by women in Facebook profiles are often strategically manipulated, if not enhanced, to focus on only the most flattering photos. The accompanying interactive discussion threads focus on physical appearance, exercise, and eating habits. Taken together, this environment is one that facilitates body comparison and leads to dissatisfaction with body image in much the same way as with conventional media exposure.

The pervasiveness of the media means that it is an agent of socialization (see Chap. 4). The music we listen to, as well as the shows and movies we watch, depict men and women interacting. Through these depictions we learn social norms about the place of men and women in society. Similarly, popular music continues to include lyrics that foster male stereotypes. These stereotypes include the idea that "real" men must possess sexual prowess and should be sexually aggressive. By contrast, "real" women should be passive sexual objects, or worse, sexual playthings for men. These confining stereotypes have far reaching implications that not only foster the continuation of traditional gender roles in the home and workplace, but continue to normalize sexual violence against women. (terBogt et al. 2010) From a public health perspective, the portrayal of sexuality in mass media is largely devoid of safe sex practices and normalizes casual and unprotected sex in a virtual world where STIs and pregnancy are nonexistent. This creates increased pressure for parents, educators, and public health professionals to work to counteract these unsafe media images.

5.10 Evolution and Human Culture

Sociology has been reticent to embrace the important advances in evolutionary theory and human behavior that have occurred over the past several decades. Perhaps there is a fear that embracing evolution would mean a resurgence of those arguments suggesting that social hierarchies of race, gender, and class are inevitable and a result of natural selection. Sociologists today refute these pseudoscientific theories that have wrongly insisted race and class inequalities were biological based. Instead, contemporary evolutionary sociology applies the Darwinian evolutionary approach to understanding culture.

Cultural evolution, also called sociocultural evolution, describes the forces that explain stability and change in human culture over time. Sociologists Patrick Nolan and Gerhard Lenski (2015) describe the three forces that influence cultural evolution. The first is *continuity*, the tendency for social arrangements to remain stable over time unless interrupted by some event or innovation. The second force is *innovation*, which is also inevitable and sometimes acts to disrupt the current social arrangements. Finally, there is the force of *selection*, which determines which cultural elements survive or are eliminated.

In general, cultural elements of society are remarkably stable. Think about it, the basic structure of many elements of society, like the family, religion, a governing body of some sort, the use of written communication, art, and even a system of time have remained relatively consistent for thousands of years. The persistence of many cultural elements (art, the family, religion) may be explained by the fact that they fulfill personal needs. Social change can also be prevented by groups in power, who will act to preserve their own power in society. Innovations that are likely to disrupt the social order are prevented or controlled by powerful groups who strive to maintain their power. Another force for stability, or continuity, is socialization. Societies have a remarkable ability to sustain culture over time, generation to generation through **socialization** (for a definition and more details, see Chap. 4). This process of passing culture down from generation to generation is called **cultural transmission**. Just as individuals pass their genes from one generation to the next through sexual reproduction, societies pass culture down from one society to the next through the socialization process in which language, norms, and values are transmitted from one generation to the next.

Despite the many forces acting to maintain stability, there are also disruptive forces that occur. Technological inventions like the automobile, the airplane, and the television are inventions that exert pressure for social change. The birth control pill is another important example of an invention that has had major influence on gender roles in society. Not only do changes occur through innovations and inventions intended to solve problems, but social changes also occur as cultures come into contact with other cultures. In an increasingly global society, the opportunities to share information, inventions, and tools, from one society to the next are ever-expanded and are an important force for cultural change. The process in which one society passes material and non-material culture to another is referred to as **cultural**

diffusion. An excellent example of cultural diffusion is the incredible popularity of yoga, meditation, and mindfulness practice in American society. Not long ago, it would be unthinkable to a medical doctor to prescribe meditation or other mindfulness practices to reduce a patient's blood pressure. But, that is exactly what is happening now as a result of cultural diffusion.

In any society, there is a relatively high rate of innovations, any of which *could* result in social change, but not all do. In other words, society is often faced with a number of choices that will determine whether some invention, or other type of innovation is embraced and becomes the basis for social change. When members of a society embrace an innovation that results in large scale social change, they are essentially making a choice. The invention of the automobile created a car culture in the U.S. that changed not only transportation, but how and where we live. In a sense, embracing the automobile, and casting off the horse and buggy is an example of the selection process. This type of selection occurs within a society. But, there are other ways selection happens too. Another type of selection occurs when two or more societies are engaged in competition for territory. Consider the indigenous societies in the United States, Canada, and Australia, among others. The European settlers possessed more advanced technology, had greater numbers, and a more complex social organization. These characteristics amounted to advantages that resulted in the effective dissolution of indigenous cultures. In some cases, entire cultures essentially disappeared, in other cases, as with indigenous societies, certain elements of the culture remain, but the societies are changed forever.

It's important to keep in mind that since nearly all societies include powerful groups of elites (see Chap. 9) the selection processes that occur in cultural evolution do not always select the most adaptive innovations. Rather, sometimes the selection process can occur as a result of groups in power making choices that benefit themselves; sometimes to the detriment of the broader social order. The rapid expansion of the fast food industry throughout the world, for example, is certainly an example of maladaptive cultural evolution which is the result of large and powerful corporate interests. There is little question that the expansion of fast food has resulted in large scale cultural changes. It can also be regarded as maladaptive to the extent that it is partially responsible for an increasing obesity epidemic. Unlike biological evolution, in which adaption is a central mechanism for selection, cultural evolution is under human control and as such is not strictly speaking analogous to biological evolution.

Key Terms and Definitions

- **Social Norms** (Content Category 7B): unspoken rules that guide our day-to-day behavior.
  - **Sanctions**: penalties used to enforce norms.
  - **Rewards**: A positive sanction, used to reinforce norms.
  - **Folkways**: social norms involving etiquette that carry very light penalties.
  - **Mores**: social norms with a moral component.
  - **Taboos**: norm that carries a strong moral component whose violation caries severe punishment.

- **Ethnocentrism** (Content Category 8B): the tendency to look down on other cultures, and judge them using your own cultural standards.
- **Cultural relativism**: the opposite of ethnocentrism and means judging a culture by its own standards.

  Elements of Culture (Content Category 9A)
- **Culture**: nearly every aspect of our day-to-day lives. It includes our values and rules that govern our behavior, our language, the way we dress, our tools and technology, music, art, and religion.
  - **Material Culture**: physical objects such as tools, art, and clothing; symbolic, or non-material culture includes beliefs, values, and norms.
- **Beliefs**: ideas about what is true.
- **Values**: abstract ideas about what is desirable or not desirable, right or wrong, good or bad.
- **Rituals**: group activities or actions, often performed at specific times and places that serve to unite individuals around culturally important values.
- **Symbols**: objects or images that convey meaning, and often represent cultural beliefs.
  - **Language**: system of symbols that allows humans to communicate.
- **Culture Lag**: a situation where social norms are disrupted by rapid social and technological change.
- **Culture Shock**: the personal confusion and discomfort that is felt when being confronted with an unfamiliar culture.
- **Cultural Evolution**: also called sociocultural evolution, describes the forces that explain stability and change in human cultures over time.
- **Cultural Transmission**: process of transferring culture from one generation to the next.
- **Cultural Diffusion**: process of transferring culture from one society to another.
- **Assimilation**: adopting the cultural elements, the values, norms, language, dress and traditions of the dominant culture of the host country.
- **Multiculturalism**: acknowledging, accepting, and celebrating diverse cultures equally.
- **Subcultures**: groups with unique norms, values, and language that sets them apart from mainstream society.
- **Counterculture** a special type of subculture whose norms, values and attitudes are in direct conflict or opposition to mainstream culture.
- **Mass Media**: all forms of mass communication designed to reach large anonymous audiences including newspapers, radio, television, movies, streaming video, and internet sources such as websites, blogs, and social media.
- **Popular Culture**: the mass-produced ideas, images and entertainment designed to be accessible to a large audience.

Activities and Research Examples

Activity 1: Subcultures.

What subcultures are you a part of? Identify one or more social groups that you are involved in and ask yourself if these would be considered subcultures. Do these groups have unique norms or language?

Activity 2: Media Influence.

Carefully observe and reflect on the images that you see on television, movies, music videos or the internet. You can make a journal to record these observations. What kinds of messages do you see about healthy and unhealthy behaviors? How might these messages influence young audiences?

Resources, Links, and Recommended Readings

Recommended reading for culture in health care.

Fadiman, Anne. (1998) *The spirit catches you and you fall down: a Hmong child, her American doctors, and the collision of two cultures* New York: Noonday Press.

Recommended resources for mass media.

Herman, E. S., & Chomsky, N. (2010). Manufacturing consent: The political economy of the mass media. Random House.
Kilbourne, J. (2002). Killing Us Softly 3 (FILM): Advertising's Image of Women.

Culture and Language. The Linguistic Society of America's Culture and Language website includes resources and recommended readings on a broad range of topics related to linguistic relativity and determinism. http://www.linguisticsociety.org/resource/language-and-thought

The Think Cultural Health website includes interactive maps and testimonials by health care providers about providing culturally and linguistically appropriate services (CLAS). It also includes free e-learning modules related to CLAS. https://cccm.thinkculturalhealth.hhs.gov/

A culturally relevant guide to Native American ceremonial tobacco use can be found at http://keepitsacred.itcmi.org/

Critical Media Project. The Critical Media Project is designed to serve educators who "seek to incorporate media literacy into the classroom. This site contains a wide range of media artifacts that explore the politics of identity across issues of race, ethnicity and glass, gender, and sexuality." http://www.criticalmediaproject.org/cml/topicbackground/race-ethnicity/

The Centers for Disease Control National Health Interview Survey Website includes a whole host of interactive data tables related to health behaviors and health. **https://www.cdc.gov/nchs/nhis/index.htm**

The Kaiser Family Foundation website includes health policy brief documents designed to provide up-to-date information on a host of health policy issues. The Health Coverage and Care for Immigrants issue brief explains the current Affordable Care Act rules about providing health care to immigrant populations. **http://www.kff.org/disparities-policy/issue-brief/health-coverage-and-care-for-immigrants/**

Study Questions

1. **Define the term culture. What are the related concepts?**
2. **How does culture connect to health?**

***Example Exam Question:** "The use of prominent warning labels on cigarette packs best supports which statement?

A. The social stigma of risky health behaviors decreases with age.
B. Peer pressure is the primary motivator in reducing health risks.
C. Tolerance of risky health behaviors has increased over time.
D. Social norms about health risks are enforced through sanctions." (AAMC 2012: 117)

*For more information, visit https://students-residents.aamc.org/applying-medical-school/article/whats-mcat-exam/

References

Association of American Medical Colleges (AAMC). (2011). *Preview guide for the MCAT 2015 exam*. www.aamc.org/MCAT2015.

Association of American Medical Colleges (AAMC). (2012). *Preview guide for the MCAT 2015 exam* (2nd ed.). www.aamc.org/MCAT2015.

Association of American Medical Colleges (AAMC). (2015). *The official guide to the MCAT exam (MCAT2015)* (4th ed.). Washington, DC: The Association of American Medical Colleges.

Cohen, R., & Blaszczynski, A. (2015). Comparative effects of Facebook and conventional media on body image dissatisfaction. *J Eating Disorders, 3*, 23.

Dixon, T. L., & Linz, D. (2000). Overrepresentation and underrepresentation of American Americans and Latinos as lawbreakers on television news. *Journal of Communication, 50*(2), 131–154.

Evans, W. N., Farrelly, M. C., & Montgomery, E. (1999). Do workplace bans reduce smoking? *The American Economic Review, 89*(4), 728–747.

Friedlander, W. J. (1992). *The golden wand of medicine: A history of the Caduceus symbol in medicine*. New York: Greenwood Press. ISBN 0-313-28023-1.

Herman, E. S., & Chomsky, N. (2010). *Manufacturing consent: The political economy of the mass media*. Random House.

Hersch, J. (2017). Skin color, immigrant wages, and discrimination. In R. Hall (Ed.), *Racism in the 21st century* (pp. 77–90). New York: Springer.

LaVeist, T. A. (2012). *Race, ethnicity, and health: A public health reader* (p. 848). San Francisco: Jossey-Bass.

Nolan, P., & Lenski, G. (2015). *Human societies* (10th ed.). Boulder: Paradigm Publishers.

PwC. (2016). *The wearable life 2.0: Connected living in a wearable world*. https://www.pwc.com/us/en/industry/entertainment-media/assets/pwc-cis-wearables.pdf

Rabin, R. C. (2010). Respecting Muslim patient's needs. *New York Times*. http://www.nytimes.com/2010/11/01/health/01patients.html?_r=0

terBogt, T. F. M., Engels, R. C. M. E., Bogers, S., et al. (2010). Shake it baby shake it: Media preferences, sexual attitudes and gender stereotypes among adolescents. *Sex Roles, 63*, 844. doi:10.1007/s11199-010-9815-1.

The Harris Poll. (2016). *Tattoo takeover: Three in ten Americans have tattoos, and most don't stop at just one*, @HarrisPoll. http://www.theharrispoll.com/health-and-life/Tattoo_Takeover.html

U.S. Department of Health and Human Services (USDHHS). (2017). Be tobacco free.Gov http://betobaccofree.hhs.gov/laws/

Chapter 6
Race and Ethnicity

Objectives

- Introduce and define race and ethnicity
- Differentiate between prejudice and discrimination and identify their sources
- Provide a historical overview of racism
- Examine the connection between race/ethnicity and health outcomes
- Develop ability to effectively communicate and collaborate with individuals with various backgrounds

Foundational Concept 8
"*Psychological, sociocultural, and biological factors influence the way we think about ourselves and others.*" (AAMC 2012: 107)

Category 8B (*attitudes and beliefs that effect social interactions*) focuses on attitudes and beliefs that affect social interactions including prejudice, bias, and stereotyping.

"Social thinking refers to the ways in which we view others and our environment, as well as how we interpret others' behaviors. A variety of factors – personality, environment, and culture – factor into the beliefs and attitudes we develop" (AAMC 2012: 107)

Category 8C (*social interactions*) focuses on the actions and processes underlying social interactions and discrimination.

"Human beings are social by nature. Though the sentiment is simple, the actions and processes underlying and shaping our social interactions are not" (AAMC 2012: 108)

G. Garcia-Alexander et al., *Social Foundations of Behavior for the Health Sciences*,
DOI 10.1007/978-3-319-64950-4_6

6.1 Connecting Health to Race and Ethnicity

At present, researchers and policy makers are in agreement that racial and ethnic disparities in health are widespread and persistent in the U.S. What this means in real life is persistently poorer outcomes among racial and ethnic minorities across several health and health care measures. For example, African Americans, American Indians, and Latinos generally report barriers to accessing care and poorer quality of care than whites. In addition, African Americans are more likely to experience late stage diagnoses (ex. advanced breast cancer), have higher rates of maternal death, and have higher rates of diabetes (AHRQ 2014). In addition, they experience higher rates of mortality across many of the most common causes of death in the U.S. Despite numerous efforts to investigate these differences and identify their sources, we remain largely unable to pinpoint their exact source or how best to reduce them. Racial and ethnic disparities in health may be attributable to personal characteristics (level of education, class status, occupational status, etc.), environmental factors (e.g. unhealthy/unsafe neighborhoods), differences in access to care, provider-level factors (differential treatment and recommendations), and/or system-evel factors (public policies related to Medicaid/Medicare and privatization of medicine). Nonetheless, the health care community is committed to reducing and ultimately removing racial and ethnic health disparities. A related point to recognize is that it's difficult to disentangle race and ethnicity from social class. In other words, minorities are more likely to have lower socio-economic status than whites in the U.S. This too contributes to poorer health outcomes.

Throughout this chapter, we will explore our ideas about what race really is, how it's a socially constructed concept, and how it contributes to poorer outcomes in some groups relative to others. In addition, we will consider racism at the individual and institutional levels, prejudice, stereotyping, and discrimination. Various studies have shown the impact of racism and stereotyping in leading to disparate health outcomes. In addition, factors at the system level (meaning policies and structural mechanisms) can also lead to poorer health outcomes. As health professionals, it's imperative to be aware of the influences of such factors. In addition, it's a necessity to be self-reflective and aware of any biases that may endanger an effective patient-provider alliance.

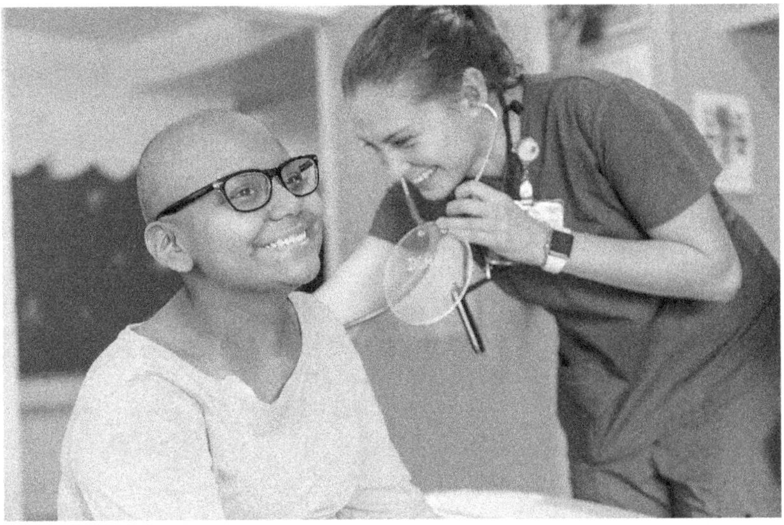

Patient-provider interaction (Source: OHSU Digital Commons, https://www.ohsu.edu/custom/library/digital-collections/files/original/66ce1c73ab4d7e5073237e2beb084fc0.jpg)

6.2 A Sociological Understanding of Race and Ethnicity

Sociologists see race as a socially constructed category that's based on physical criteria. The **social construction of race** refers to the argument that racial differences are not biological, but are instead based on social ideas about what it means to belong to one race group versus another. In fact, the genes that determine skin color have no connection to intelligence, athletic ability, or musical talent. The shared ideas we as a society have about what it means to belong to one group or another are passed on through the socialization process and have deep historical roots. Sociologists emphasize these historical processes that occur at the individual and institutional level and ultimately lead to our understanding of race today. Thus, racial divides are not based on inherent physical differences but on socially constructed ideas. Formally, **race** can be defined as a **socially constructed** category based on physical characteristics, i.e. skin color, hair type, etc., which distinguish it from other groups. Current racial designations in the US include White, Black or African American, American Indian/Alaska Native, Asian Indian, and others (see Fig. 6.1). It is very important to recognize that we as a society attach significance to the concept of race – thus, *the fact that we believe there are race-based differences leads to real race-based divisions in society*. To better understand how this works, let's consider the arbitrary nature of racial classifications throughout American history. If we examine the racial categories used by the census bureau, we can observe how group membership and definitions have changed over time (see Fig. 6.2). Note that these differences occurred purely in response to shifts in thought as a society not to actual changes in groups.

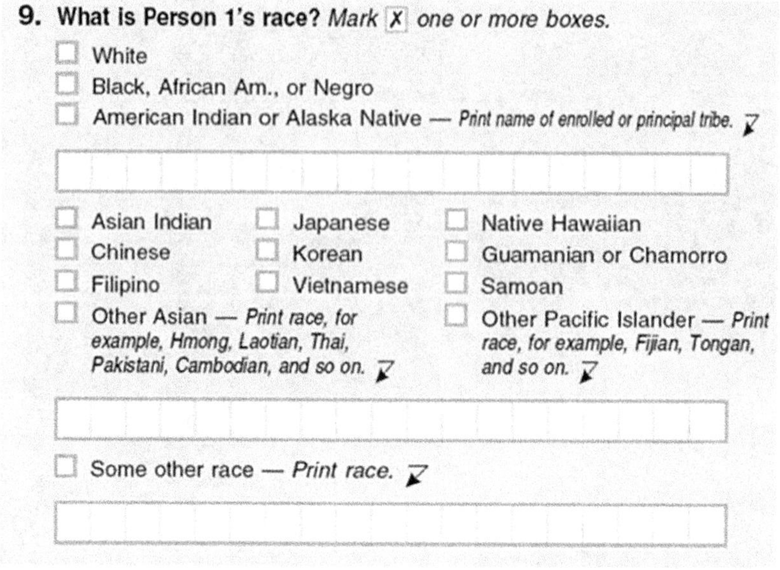
9. What is Person 1's race? Mark X one or more boxes.

- ☐ White
- ☐ Black, African Am., or Negro
- ☐ American Indian or Alaska Native — *Print name of enrolled or principal tribe.*
- ☐ Asian Indian
- ☐ Chinese
- ☐ Filipino
- ☐ Other Asian — *Print race, for example, Hmong, Laotian, Thai, Pakistani, Cambodian, and so on.*
- ☐ Japanese
- ☐ Korean
- ☐ Vietnamese
- ☐ Native Hawaiian
- ☐ Guamanian or Chamorro
- ☐ Samoan
- ☐ Other Pacific Islander — *Print race, for example, Fijian, Tongan, and so on.*
- ☐ Some other race — *Print race.*

Fig. 6.1 2010 Census race options (Source: U.S. Census Bureau; Accessed at: http://www.pewresearch.org/fact-tank/2015/06/18/census-considers-new-approach-to-asking-about-race-by-not-using-the-term-at-all/2010censusrace-2/)

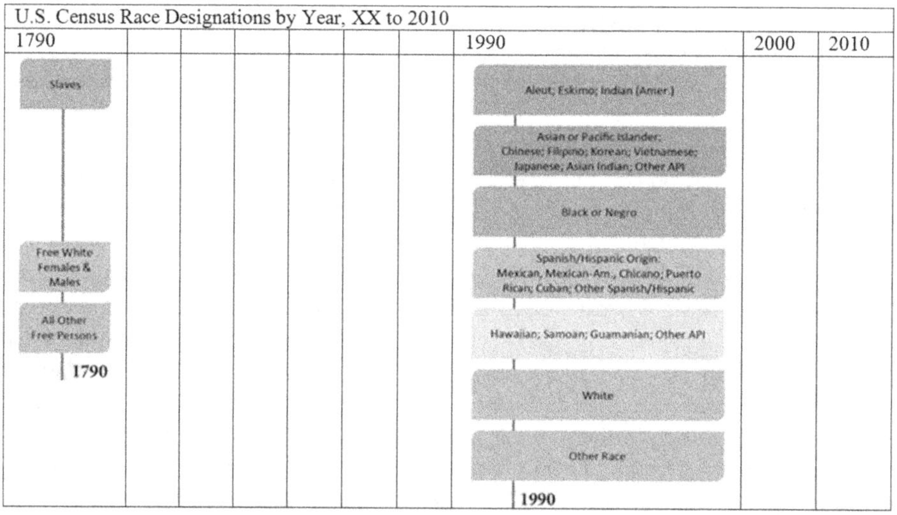

Fig. 6.2 Census categories over time (Source: Beverly M. Pratt, Lindsay Hixson, and Nicholas A. Jones. 2015. "MEASURING RACE AND ETHNICITY ACROSS THE DECADES, 1790–2010," Population Division, U.S. Census Bureau. http://www.census.gov/population/race/data/MREAD_1790_2010.html); Link to interactive infographic from census: http://www.census.gov/population/race/data/MREAD_1790_2010.html

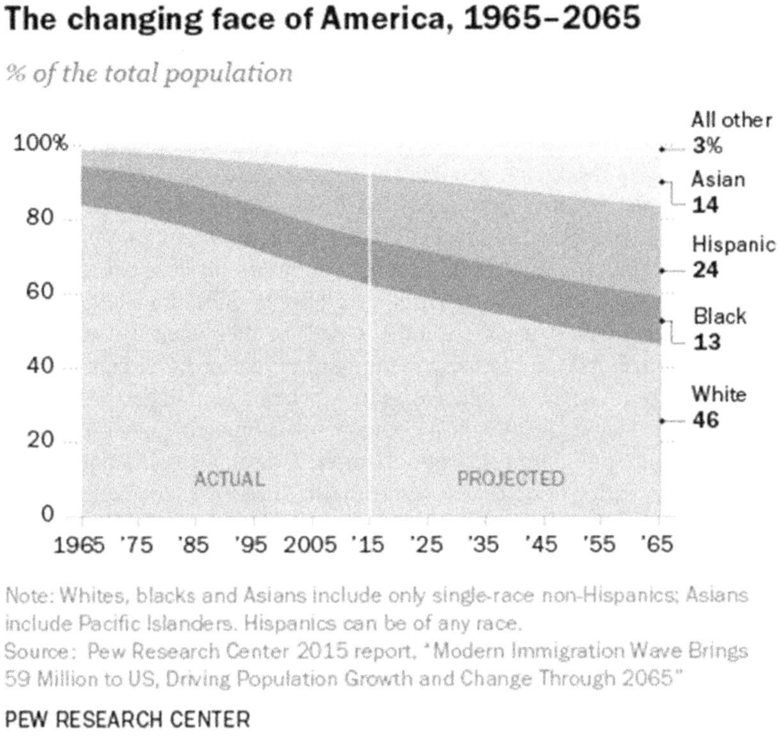

Fig. 6.3 Racial and ethnic projections in the U.S. (source: http://www.pewresearch.org/fact-tank/2016/03/31/10-demographic-trends-that-are-shaping-the-u-s-and-the-world/)

Another important concept is **ethnicity**. In contrast to race, ethnicity refers to a social category of people who share a common culture. In the United States, the only ethnicity that is officially designated on the census is used to distinguish Hispanics or Latinos. This group is technically a **pan-ethnicity**, which means it is a group that is comprised of a multitude of ethnicities. Thus, the term Latino is used to describe people from South America, Mexico, Puerto Rico, Spain, and Central America, among others. This is the largest minority group in the U.S., and they currently account for 18% of the total population (~53 million); though it is projected that there will be no racial or ethnic majority by 2055 (see Fig. 6.3) (PEW 2015).

As mentioned above, Hispanics or Latinos are what we consider a pan-ethnicity. Thus, there is a great deal of variation within the larger group. In order to effectively understand and meet the needs of and provide effective services to this diverse and growing group, one should understand some basic facts (more information on group membership is provided in Ch. 8: Demographic Structure). Hispanics or Latinos are currently comprised of a mixture of U.S. born, naturalized, and foreign-born citizens. About three-quarters are U.S. born or naturalized while the remaining quarter are foreign-born. Within Latinos, Mexicans are the largest origin group (64.1% of all Latinos in the US), followed by: Puerto Ricans, Cubans, Salvadorans, and

Dominicans (PEW 2015). Approximately 68% of Latinos report English as their only language spoken at home (or that they speak it very well) (PEW 2015). Finally, the terms Latino and Hispanic can generally be used interchangeably and most show no real preference for one term versus another. However, recent survey reports suggest that if given the option, most prefer to be identified by their country of origin, i.e. Guatemalan, Mexican, Venezuelan, etc.

Formally, ethnic minority groups are those who: (1) experience exclusion from the dominant group, (2) membership is ascribed (i.e. not by choice) rather than achieved, and (3) the members feel a sense of community. In sociology, we further distinguish between situational and symbolic ethnicity. Situational ethnicity is when a person chooses whether to assert some aspect of their identity or heritage in a particular context. For example, someone might reveal or hide their heritage on a job application. Similarly, symbolic ethnicity is when a person has fully assimilated into the dominant culture, and only participates in ethnic customs on special occasions. For example, one might actively claim their heritage as Irish on St. Patrick's Day. The key difference to note with respect to both of these concepts in relation to an ethnic minority group is the ability to choose whether or not one asserts membership in a particular group. Mary C. Waters has written on this topic and reports that an important aspect of symbolic ethnicity is that it is voluntary. She also indicates that this represents the best of all worlds for white ethnics. For more information on this topic, see the recommended reading: "Optional Ethnicities: For Whites Only?"

The United States is considered a multi-ethnic society. This means that we are comprised of a variety of racial, ethnic, religious, and cultural groups. Unlike many other societies, we allow a great deal of movement and encourage freedom of expression. Globally, the U.S. ranks as a "high diversity" society. Other countries ranked highly on diversity include Canada and Australia. On the other hand, countries such as Finland and Japan have a very low degree of diversity. With respect to how such groups become integrated with the dominant culture, there are two primary models: (1) assimilation and (2) accommodation. **Assimilation** is also referred to as the *melting pot model*, as it reflects the notion that new groups that enter U.S. society will become fully absorbed by the dominant culture. This model dictates conformity with the dominant group. On the other hand, **accommodation**, or the *salad bowl model*, encourages expression of diverse cultures and the existence of a various set of diverse cultures is accepted. This is more of an ideal than the reality in the U.S.; nonetheless, it is important to be aware of what represents **diversity** and develop a vocabulary in **cultural sensitivity** (for more information see Chap. 5: Culture).

A vast array of different groups co-exist in the United States. These groups each have their own set of norms and practices that distinguish them from other groups. Thus, the term **diversity** can be used to describe societies that are characterized by the presence of a variety of groups with distinct cultural characteristics. The term diversity may refer to race, ethnicity, national origin, sexuality, religion, and other characteristics. With respect to health care delivery, state and federal regulations encourage or may require a level of responsiveness to the increasing diversity of the U.S. population. These standards dictate that culturally and linguistically appropriate care is provided to various minority groups. For more information on federal standards see the US DHHS Standards for Culturally and Linguistically Appropriate Services at: https://www.thinkculturalhealth. hhs.gov/clas.

We are all raised/socialized with the norms of the group to which we belong. This leads us to recognize and identify patterns of behavior we are familiar with as "normal," while those we are not familiar with are seen as abnormal or are difficult for us to accept. For example, we may not feel comfortable with women wearing headscarves, or hijabs, which is a name for the dress worn by some women of Middle Eastern origin (*hijab* is the term for a head and neck cover that leaves the face clear, *niqab* refers to a scarf which reveals only the eyes, and a *burka* refers to a full cover which leaves only a mesh screen for the eyes). Indeed, the wearing of such clothing led to intense debate in France, which was sparked when three Muslim girls were suspended from school after refusing to remove their veils and ultimately led to the development of a law forbidding the wearing of "ostentatious" religious articles in school. This debate has come to be known as the "veil affair." More recently, a law that bans wearing full-face coverings in public spaces was passed due to concerns of national security (for more info see: http://www.huffingtonpost.com/news/france-burqa-ban/).

Formally, when we judge the culture or cultural practices of others based on our own standards we are engaging in **ethnocentrism**. As sociologists, we strive to recognize the importance of seeing things from another point of view. Thus, judging another's culture or cultural practices based on its own standards is referred to as **cultural relativism**. As health professionals, it is important to become familiar with these various sets of standards as they may lead to differences in health-related behaviors and beliefs. By developing familiarity, a better standard of care may be provided that is based on a shared understanding of treatment and goals (also see Chap. 5: Culture) (Box 6.1)

Box 6.1: Further Thought. Cultural Awareness and Sensitivity

Delivering care in a respectful and understandable way is key to providing quality care. Providers can also improve quality by implementing multidisciplinary treatment teams and encouraging patient education and activation in medically underserved groups. It is important to recognize that cultural sensitivity training that is not well done can have a negative effect and work to increase stereotyping. Thus, providers and other health workers should strive to familiarize themselves with the community they serve and get to know information about social and historical context, socioeconomic status, immigration experiences, healing practices, and disease prevalence (Smedley et al. 2002). For more information and training opportunities see the links and resources section.

Which groups will you serve in your practice? What norms and practices should you be familiar with? How might these impact the delivery of care and/or understanding of treatment recommendations?

6.3 Racism

As health professionals, it's necessary to learn about the historical context of racism. Formally, **racism** is defined as a system of domination that operates in social processes and social institutions; it is used to justify the unequal distribution of society's rewards. In the United States, we have a long history of racism. In the early twentieth century, racist beliefs and attitudes were supported by the science of the day. Thus, in the social sciences we have identified scientific racism, in which "scientific" evidence was compiled to promote arguments that certain groups were genetically inferior. Accordingly, Darwinism was adapted into social Darwinism. The main idea behind this concept was that some groups were unable to be assimilated into a complex, white civilization given their primitive origins. In many cases, the medical community provided support for arguments suggesting inferiority of the black race.

The scientific support provided by professionals in various disciplines in the early 1900s was an expression of **overt racism**. This means that racism was freely and openly communicated against racial minorities. Examples of overt racism included the practice of preventing blacks from purchasing land and working in certain occupations, the practice of slavery itself, and Jim Crow laws (racial separation/segregation laws enacted from 1890s to 1950s; link to timeline of events of Jim Crow era: http://www.pbs.org/wnet/jimcrow/stories_events.html). More generally,

Box 6.2: Further Thought Tuskegee Syphilis Study (for more information see: Bad Blood: The Tuskegee Syphilis Experiment by James H. Jones 1993)

In perhaps one of the most egregious acts in American public health, the U.S. Public Health Service (USPHS) withheld treatment to African American men who had syphilis in order to study the long term effects of the disease (Brandt 1978). In 1932, the USPHS initiated an experiment in Macon County, AL which observed 400 syphilitic men (an additional 200 uninfected men served as controls). The express purpose of the experiment was to observe the natural course of untreated syphilis. In exchange for participation, subjects were given access to treatment for their "bad blood," (which is what they were led to believe they were being treated for) and were offered burial services. The experiment itself was fueled by racist thoughts surrounding the sexual nature of African Americans and their propensity to seek treatment, and it is thus highly important to place it in historical context (Brandt 1978). Even after penicillin became available in the 1950s, the men were not given treatment. In fact, USPHS actively sought to prevent the men from receiving the recommended therapy. The experiment was not officially ended until 1972 when the national press became aware of its existence.

this type of racism encompasses the active prevention of certain groups from accessing certain goods and services, and/or open use of racist terms and slurs against individuals or groups. The discipline of sociology can also be critiqued for its perpetuation of racism, and several scholars point out racism was a regular part of the discipline throughout this time (for an excellent contemporary review and discussion of racism in sociology see the *Social Problems* issue listed in the *Resources, Links, and Recommended Readings* Section). In the United States, our history involves multiple instances of attempts to concentrate wealth, power, and privilege in whites, which has led to measureable gaps in education, professional success, and health outcomes in various minority groups. A more extreme example is explored in the *Further Thought* section on the Tuskegee Syphilis Experiment.

After the 1950s in the U.S., we saw a shift toward less overt forms of racism. This is often referred to **symbolic racism**, which suggests that we have shifted from the belief that groups are biologically inferior to ideas that they are culturally inferior. Symbolic racism is characterized by subtle, yet persistent stereotyping (which is often perpetuated by the media), and a tendency to argue that gaps in education or income are the result of problems inherent to some groups. A related term is **color-blind racism**. This is when individuals ignore the presence of racial inequalities. It's problematic because ignoring real differences or barriers encountered by some groups perpetuates inequalities by removing the ability to address and correct such issues. Importantly, some scholars argue that though the form of racism has changed over time, it still results in practices that achieve the same purpose, i.e. maintaining the racial status quo. They argue that the racial order was maintained during the era of slavery with physical practices (whipping/overseers), with strict written laws regarding racial contact in the Jim Crow era, and with sophisticated and subtle practices (the use of state agencies such as the criminal justice system) in this era "new racism" (Bonilla-Silva 2014). This is discussed in more detail in the section below on *institutional racism.*

The larger term *racism* encompasses two separate concepts: **prejudice** and **discrimination**. As sociologists, we distinguish between the thoughts and beliefs that contribute to racism and the actions. Thus, prejudice refers to the widely held ideas and *attitudes* about the character and ability of certain groups. Prejudice is characterized by: the presence of categorical thoughts, i.e. those about groups rather than individual or personal attributes, inflexible definitions of some groups, generally negative feelings about some groups, and stereotypes. **Stereotypes** refer to an oversimplified set of *beliefs* about members of various minority groups. They work to reinforce negative feelings about minority groups and justify the unequal treatment experienced by members of those groups. Stereotypes continue to be quite widespread in the media. Similarly, stigma is a deeply discrediting attribute that disqualifies a person from full social acceptance (Goffman 1963). Ethnicity can be thought of as a sociocultural condition that is stigmatized and leads to marginalization.

Discrimination can be motivated by prejudice and stereotyping and refers to actions or *differential treatment* of ethnic minority groups ranging from avoidance to denial or services to threats and/or physical attack. In today's society, outright prejudice and discrimination are condemned, but there is considerable evidence that they continue to be a widespread issue. In fact, in a recent survey, 46% of African Americans, 25% of Hispanics, and 16% of whites reported a lot of discrimination against African Americans (Doherty 2013). However, today's discrimination is subtle (harder to measure) and involves both verbal and nonverbal cues in social interactions. This form is sometimes referred to as *aversive racism* and often involves those who consciously endorse principles of racial equality. While the participants regard themselves as racially egalitarian, and certainly do not express open hostility toward minorities, their unconscious biases are reflected by discomfort and avoidance (Dovidio et al. 2008). Research in this area suggests that this type of discrimination is minimal in situations with well-defined standards of behavior, but it tends to increase in situations that require flexibility or judgment calls, which activates negative stereotypes (Dovidio and Gaertner 2000). For example, in a study of hiring practices it was observed that there was little evidence of discrimination if applicants were highly qualified or poorly qualified. However, if there was uncertainty with respect to the level of skill, participants more commonly favored a white applicant versus a black applicant (Dovidio and Gaertner 2000; Pager and Shepherd 2008). Similar evidence has been observed in the healthcare setting and has indicated that disparities in treatment are more common in scenarios that require discretion, i.e. referrals or testing. Additionally, this form is communicated via nonverbal cues of discrimination including eye contact (or lack thereof) and body language.

For the most part we have considered racism at the individual level, but it can also occur at the institutional level. **Institutional discrimination, or institutional racism,** is that which is built into the structure of a society and acts in a systematic way to create barriers and unequal access to services. For example, the fact that minorities have a harder time getting a home loan or are imprisoned at rates far higher than non-Hispanic whites, is evidence of institutional discrimination. In the healthcare setting, it has become well-accepted that this plays an important role in the production of health disparities. In *Unequal Treatment* (2002) a comprehensive report published by the Institutes of Medicine (IOM), these are referred to as system-level factors are shown to exert a measureable impact on the quality of care and health outcomes. Thus, various aspects of the system itself (reimbursement procedures, geographic availability, and managed care) may create barriers for minority patients. The IOM reports,

> Complicated reimbursement procedures and structures…may deter patients with low literacy or limited English proficiency from seeking care. Similarly, time pressures on physicians may hamper the ability of providers to accurately assess presenting symptoms of minority patients…rapid changes in the financing and delivery of healthcare services – such as the dramatic shifts brought by cost-control efforts and the movement to managed care – may pose greater barriers for racial and ethnic minorities than for non-minorities (2002: 140).

In an excellent example developed by Camara Jones (2000), one can easily understand the impacts of racism and how it operates at the individual versus the institutional level (Fig. 6.4). In this example, two flower pots are used to represent the experiences of different groups. One pot is filled with soil from the previous season and the other is empty. The gardener fills the empty pot with fresh soil and leaves

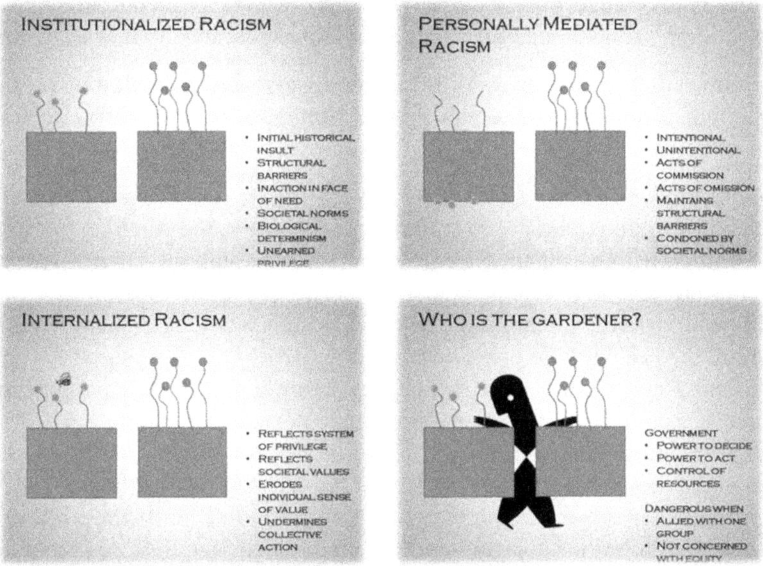

Fig. 6.4 Images adapted from: Levels of racism: A theoretic framework and a gardener's tale (Available at: http://www.ncbi.nlm.nih.gov/pmc/articles/PMC1446334/pdf/10936998.pdf)

the other pot as is, then sows different colored seeds in each of the two. The seeds planted in the new soil grow quickly and flourish, while the seeds planted in the old soil struggle and do not grow as large. The pots depict institutional or structural disadvantages that are built into the system. Accordingly, this is powerful imagery that can be used to effectively depict the importance of the presence of institutionalized racism. People have access to different resources which translate into differences in their access to quality education, safe and clean environments to live and work in, high quality health facilities, and so on; this naturally impacts their entire lives.

Going back to the example, the gardener may choose to plant their favorite colored seed in the box with the fresh soil. They may then go on to add plant food and actively cultivate this crop (because it's their favorite colored flower) and leave the other alone. This active preference for one colored flower versus the other represents personally mediated racism, or prejudice and discrimination, as described above. It may take the form of failure to provide service, surprise at someone's competence, or more extreme forms, like hate crimes. Finally, the gardener represents the government, since ultimately it controls the resources and sets the tone for how discrimination is addressed formally.

Key Terms and Definitions

- **Race** (Content Category 9B): a socially constructed category based on physical characteristics that distinguish group members
  - Social construction of race:

- **Ethnicity**: a category of people who share a common culture; in the U.S., Hispanic or Latino is the only officially designated ethnicity
  - Ethnic minority groups are those that display unique cultural traits, suffer prejudice and discrimination by the dominant group, and membership is ascribed
- **Assimilation** (Content Category 9A): distinctive ethnic group features are absorbed into dominant group culture; also known as the "melting pot model"
- **Accommodation** (Content Category 9A): diverse cultural features and characteristics are accepted in society; also known as the "salad bowl model"
- **Ethnocentrism** (Content Category 8B): a tendency to judge other groups or cultures on the standards of one's own culture
- **Cultural Relativism** (Content Category 8B): the belief that the concepts and values of a culture must be understood in context
- **Cultural Competence**: the ability of individuals and systems to respond respectfully and effectively to people of all cultures, classes, races, ethnic backgrounds, and religions in a manner that recognizes, affirms, and values the cultural differences and similarities and the worth of individuals, families, and communities (source: Seattle-King County Public Health)
- **Racism**: encompasses prejudice and discrimination; the belief that one's own group is superior to others and provides support for discriminatory practices
  - **Overt**: belief that some groups are biologically inferior
  - **Covert/Symbolic**: belief that some groups are culturally inferior. Symbolic racism is characterized by subtle, yet persistent stereotyping and a tendency to argue that achievement gaps are the result of problems inherent to some groups
    - **Aversive**: more indirect and subtle form of racism that characterizes the racial attitudes of well-educated liberal whites and is activated in discretionary scenarios
  - **Color-blind**: the avoidance of racial language in an effort to suggest racism is not an issue when it actually is
- **Prejudice** (Content Category 8B): encompasses the attitudes about the character and ability of certain groups
  - **Stereotypes**: an oversimplified set of beliefs about members of various minority groups
  - **Stigma**: a characteristic or trait that sets people apart from others and results in social disapproval
- **Discrimination**: unequal/differential treatment of people or groups
  - **Individual/Interpersonal**: unequal treatment reflected in interactions between two or more people
  - **Institutional discrimination**: practices that are built into the structure of a society and act in a systematic way to create barriers and unequal access to services

Activities and Research Examples

Activity 1: IAT Test > understanding and recognizing implicit bias

The Implicit Association Test (IAT) is a tool developed by a team of researchers to measure attitudes and beliefs that people may be unwilling or unable to report. It can be an especially useful tool for uncovering implicit attitudes or stereotypes you are not aware of. A number of different tests are available on: weight, Native American, Follow the link shown to navigate to the IAT (https://implicit.harvard.edu/implicit/takeatest.html). Choose one or more of the tests to take. After completing the test, consider the results. Were they surprising to you? How can you use this information to improve your ability to interact with others and/or reduce stereotyping?

Activity 2: Awareness of stereotyping

Following the IAT test, you may now be aware of stereotypes or biases that influence your perceptions of others (for more information also see the recommended reading on racism and health). Begin a journal to keep track of your inner dialogue when you see or interact with members of this group. Consider such things as whether you have any stereotypes of minority group members, whether you express any nonverbal cues that may be interpreted/perceived as aversive racism, and what influences your feelings and beliefs about members of various groups. Also consider how these beliefs and feelings may translate into health practice (remember that perceptions of discrimination may lead to avoidance of care and internal feelings of racism/stereotypes may lead to less time spent with patients and differential recommendations). Reflect on these items and also consider ways that you might reduce or challenge any stereotypes you may have.

Activity 3: Think Cultural Health

The Department of Health and Human Services has put together several modules to help health professionals be culturally responsive and provide effective care to the diverse populations they serve. As part of this training, a module is available: *Stopping Discrimination Before it Starts*. Review the related slides and materials in the Think Cultural Health resource (link to guide and slides below) and have an in-class discussion on the impact of civil rights.

Resources, Links, and Recommended Readings

Recommended Readings on Race/Racism:

American Sociological Association. 2003. *The Importance of Collecting Data and Doing Social Scientific Research on Race*. American Sociological Association.

Bonilla-Silva, E. 2014. Racism without Racists, 4th Edition. *Colorblind Racism and the Persistence of Inequality in the United States*. New York: Rowman and Littlefield.

Essays on Voices from the Margins: Inequalities in the Sociological House. 2017. *Social Problems* 64(2), special issue.

Jones, James H. 1993. *Bad Blood: The Tuskegee Syphilis Experiment*. New York: The Free Press.

Massey, Douglas S., and Nancy A. Denton. *American Apartheid: Segregation and the Making of the Underclass*. Harvard University Press, 1993.

Unequal Treatment: What Healthcare Providers Need to Know about Racial and Ethnic Disparities in Healthcare. https://iom.nationalacademies.org/~/media/Files/Report%20Files/2003/Unequal-Treatment-Confronting-Racial-and-ethnic-Disparities-in-Health-Care/Disparitieshcproviders8pgFINAL.pdf

Waters, Mary C. 1996. "Optional Ethnicities: For Whites Only?" p. 444–54. in Silvia Pedraza and Ruben G. Rumbaut, eds. *Origins and Destines: Immigration, Race, and Ethnicity in America*. Belmont, CA: Wadsworth.

Williams DR, and Collins C. 1995. US Socioeconomic and Racial Differences in Health: Patterns and Explanations. *Annual Review of Sociology* 21:349–86.

Williams, David R. and Selina A. Mohammed. 2013. "Racism and Health I: Pathways and Scientific Evidence" *American Behavioral Scientist*, 57(8): 1152–1173.

Bias Toolkit, The RUDD Center for Food Policy and Obesity: A comprehensive toolkit developed for providers to deal with issues related to weight bias, though the tools are applicable for many stigmatized characteristics. Resources range from simple strategies to improve provider-patient communication and ways to make positive changes in the office environment, to profound ones, including self-examination of personal biases. http://biastoolkit.uconnruddcenter.org/

Healthy People 2020: Healthy People provides science-based, 10-year national objectives for improving the health of all Americans. https://www.healthypeople.gov/

Health Services Research Information Central (HSRIC): provides access to specially curated resources for high quality data and information for the health services research community. https://www.nlm.nih.gov/hsrinfo/disparities.html

Office of Minority Health: The Office of Minority Health is dedicated to improving the health of racial and ethnic minority populations through the development of health policies and programs that will help eliminate health disparities. http://minorityhealth.hhs.govv/omh/browse.aspx?lvl=2&lvlid=10

Pew Hispanic Center: provides a wealth of information on the past and current characteristics of Hispanics in the U.S. along with projections for future trends. http://www.pewhispanic.org/

Racial Equity Tools: Racial Equity Tools is designed to support individuals and groups working to achieve racial equity. This site offers tools, research, tips, curricula and ideas for people who want to increase their own understanding and to help those working toward justice at every level – in systems, organizations, communities and the culture at large. https://www.racialequitytools.org/home

The Cross Cultural Health Care Program: enacted to serve as a bridge between communities and health care institutions to advance access to quality health care that is culturally and linguistically appropriate. http://xculture.org/cultural-competency-programs/about-cultural-competency/

United States Census Bureau https://www.census.gov/

Study Questions

2. **Define the terms racism, prejudice, discrimination. What are the sources of each? How they connect to health outcomes and behaviors?**
3. **How might gender differences play a role in the healthcare setting?**

***Example Exam Question:** When health professionals change or adapt their treatment recommendations on the basis of a patient's race or ethnicity, they are engaging in:

A. Stereotyping
B. Multiculturalism
C. Claims-Making
D. Discrimination

*The above example is an author created question, please refer to https://students-residents.aamc.org/applying-medical-school/article/whats-mcat-exam/ for more information for additional sample questions and information on the entrance exam

References

Agency for Healthcare Research and Quality (AHRQ). (2014). *National Healthcare Disparities Report*, 2013. Chapter 11. Priority populations. Agency for Healthcare Research and Quality, Rockville. http://www.ahrq.gov/research/findings/nhqrdr/nhdr13/chap11.html

Association of American Medical Colleges (AAMC). (2012). *Preview guide for the MCAT 2015 exam* (2nd ed.). www.aamc.org/MCAT2015.

Bonilla-Silva, E. (2014). Racism without racists, (4th ed.). *Colorblind racism and the persistence of inequality in the United States*. New York: Rowman and Littlefield.

Brandt, A. M. (1978). Racism and research: The case of the Tuskegee syphilis study. *Hastings Center Report, 8*(6), 21–29.

Doherty, C. (2013). *For African Americans, discrimination is not dead.* In Fact Tank News in the Numbers: Pew Research Center.

Dovidio, J. F., & Gaertner, S. L. (2000). Aversive racism and selection decisions. *Psychological Science, 11*(4), 315–319.

Dovidio, J. F., Penner, L. A., Albrecht, T. L., Norton, W. E., Gaertner, S. L., & Nicole Shelton, J. (2008). Disparities and distrust: The implications of psychological processes for understanding racial disparities in health and health care. *Social Science & Medicine, 67*(3), 478–486.

Goffman, E. (1963). *Stigma: Notes on the management of spoiled identity*. New York: Simon & Schuster.

Jones, C. P. (2000). Levels of racism: A theoretic framework and a Gardener's tale. *American Journal of Public Health., 90*(8), 1212–1215.

Pager, D., & Shepherd, H. (2008). The sociology of discrimination: Racial discrimination in employment, housing, credit, and consumer markets. *Annual Review of Sociology, 34*, 181–209.

PEW Research Center. (2015). *Modern immigration wave brings 59 Million to US, driving population growth and change through 2065*. Available at: http://www.pewresearch.org/fact-tank/2016/03/31/10-demographic-trends-that-are-shaping-the-u-s-and-the-world/

Smedley, B. D., Stith, A. Y., & Nelson, A. R., (Eds.) (2002). *Unequal treatment: Confronting racial and ethnic disparities in health care*. Institute of Medicine, Committee on Understanding and Eliminating Racial and Ethnic Disparities in Health Care. Washington, DC: National Academies Press.

Chapter 7
Social Structure and Institutions

Objectives

- Describe how education reflects and reproduces culture and social inequality.
- Describe changes in family arrangements in twenty-first century.
- Describe the modernization of religion in America.
- Describe the influence of each of the social institutions on health.

> **Foundational Concept 9**
> "*Cultural and social differences influence well-being...*
> *Content Category 9A* focuses on the link between social structures and human interactions." (AAMC 2015 Pg. 255)
> "The content of this category provides a foundation for understanding social structure and the various forms of interactions within and among societies. It includes theoretical approaches to studying society and social groups, specific social institutions relevant to student preparation for medical school, and the construct of culture." (AAMC 2015 Pg. 256)

The **social structure** generally refers to the social arrangements that organize a group or society. One way to think about social structures are as hierarchies that organize our social relationships in social institutions. **Social institutions** are structures that are patterned on the basis of social needs. They include the family, education, religion, the economy, politics, and health care. These institutions are thought to fulfill societal needs, which include the replacement of membership, the socialization of members, the maintenance of social order, providing members with a sense of purpose, and the production and distribution of goods and services.

G. Garcia-Alexander et al., *Social Foundations of Behavior for the Health Sciences*,
DOI 10.1007/978-3-319-64950-4_7

7.1 Social Institutions

7.1.1 Education

Education, like the family, is a social institution charged with the task of transmitting culture and knowledge to members of society. It both reflects the culture and social arrangements of society, and serves to reinforce them. By attending public or private schools, students learn both the formal and informal curriculum. The formal curriculum provides skills and knowledge necessary to earn a living or function in society. The informal curriculum, also called the **hidden curriculum** is where norms, values, attitudes and behaviors are learned. Through interactions with administrators, teachers, and peers, students learn desirable cultural traits such as honesty, courage, punctuality, self-discipline, motivation, and obedience. Students also learn important attitudes and skills for getting along with peers including tolerance and cooperation with fellow students. Many of these traits are reinforced through a system of rewards and punishments. Other more subtle norms are also learned, though not often discussed. Students learn the proper way to interact with authority. While it may vary from culture to culture, in the U.S. elementary students learn to speak only when spoken to, raise their hand, and look the teacher in the eye when speaking. Finally, schools use a system of rewards, badges, ribbons, and certificates, for example, to develop achievement and success orientations.

One might argue that learning traditional American values and norms are helpful for getting along in society. Many sociologists, however, argue that the educational system was developed in order to create a class of obedient and achievement oriented workers with the necessary social skills and cultural values to maintain capitalist production. In fact, it is not the skills learned as part of the formal curriculum that determine future earnings, but attitudes learned through the hidden curriculum (Bowles and Gintis 1976).

The hidden curriculum also includes lessons about gender and racial stereotypes. A recent examination of elementary school learning materials, for example, showed that science textbooks more often show women as teachers, and men as scientists (Kerkhoven et al. 2016). Teachers themselves also reinforce both gender and racial stereotypes by subtly treating girls differently than boys, and treating White students differently than their minority peers. For example, teachers might call on boys, or White students more often giving the impression that they are more likely to provide correct answers.

7.1.2 Teacher Expectancy

In 1965, a Harvard social psychologist and an elementary school principal teamed up to conduct an experiment (Rosenthal and Jacobson 1968). They told a group of elementary school teachers that their students had been administered an aptitude test, and then provided them with the names of students with a high chance of success, and students with a low chance of success. Of course the test was a fake, and the students were simply randomly selected to be in the high and low achieving groups. They wanted to find out if teachers' expectations about the success of their students would affect student achievement. As you might have expected, those students whom the teachers thought were high achievers showed better academic performance than those their teachers believed would be less successful. This self-fulfilling prophecy is known as the **teacher expectancy** effect, also known as the "Pygmalion effect" in which teachers' expectations of a student or group of students affects their academic achievement. There are a number of ways that teachers' expectations may influence student performance. The students that are perceived as having more promise may get more challenging work, and also more attention and support in doing that work than those perceived to be low performers. Students also recognize when they are receiving more challenging work, more support and more positive feedback, than other students and thus work harder to achieve. This process can be described as a self-fulfilling prophecy in which teachers' attitudes and behavior influence their students' self-concept and motivation, resulting in higher performance, which in turn influences the teachers' perception of the student as a high performer (Friedrich et al. 2015).

7.1.3 Educational Segregation and Inequality

Although schools were desegregated in 1954 by a landmark Supreme Court decision in Brown v. Board of Education of Topeka, Kansas, schools remain segregated to this day. **School segregation** describes the unequal distribution of minority and White students in schools. So how segregated are America's schools today? Very segregated, in fact most White students attend schools where more than three-quarters of their fellow students are White. On the other hand, most Blacks and Hispanics attend schools where fewer than one-third are White (Orfield and Lee 2006).

Segregation continues because school boundaries still by and large coincide with neighborhood boundaries, and thus reflect the racial and economic composition of the neighborhoods. In short, schools are segregated, because they are located inside our segregated American communities. Having racially homogeneous communities would not necessarily be a problem if social and economic resources were distributed equally. However, the history of racism in society has led to racial segregation being directly tied to economic inequality. The neighborhoods in which most minorities in America live are characterized by high rates of poverty, lack of high-paying jobs, and lack of amenities like parks, grocery stores, and even movie theaters.

Shortly after the Brown v. Board of Education decision, there was a concerted effort by the federal government to integrate schools as a way to improve racial equality in education. However, since neighborhoods were segregated, the only way

Table 7.1 Racial composition of American schools

The average **White** student attends a school that is:	78% White	9% Black	9% Latino	3% Asian	1% American Indian
The average **Black** student attends a school that is:	30% White	53% Black	13% Latino	3% Asian	1% American Indian
The average **Latino** student attends a school that is:	28% White	12% Black	55% Latino	5% Asian	1% American Indian
The average **Asian** student attends a school that is:	45% White	12% Black	20% Latino	22% Asian	1% American Indian
The average **American Indian** student attends a school that is:	44% White	7% Black	11% Latino	3% Asian	35% American Indian

to integrate schools was to put minority students on buses, and send them to neighboring schools that were predominantly White. Busing was very expensive and controversial. Moving students from predominantly Black neighborhoods to predominantly White neighborhoods often increased racial tensions. Many White parents were opposed to busing their children to a poorer minority neighborhood and protested or moved their children out of public schools. By the late 1970s, the federal government began to dismantle school busing and other integration programs. Since the 1980s, there has been a process of re-segregation that has returned our school system to the highly segregated institution it is today (see Table 7.1). Although many people tend to think of segregation as an old issue from the 1960s and no longer relevant, segregation in American schools continues to present a number of challenging problems, especially for the large number of minority students who remain in segregated schools, despite the fact that evidence shows minority students are more likely to succeed academically in integrated schools (Eaton and Rivkin 2010).

7.1.4 Educational Stratification

Schools also reflect the social inequality that exists in the broader society. Schools very often derive their income from the local tax base. This means that many school districts in predominantly White communities across the county are advantaged by a richer tax base, and more funding than minority communities. In other words, education does not provide a level playing field. **Educational stratification** refers to the unequal distribution of educational resources in society. Even in states that distribute tax funds more equally across school districts, wealthier parents in high-income neighborhoods raise millions of private dollars that disproportionately benefit their own public schools.

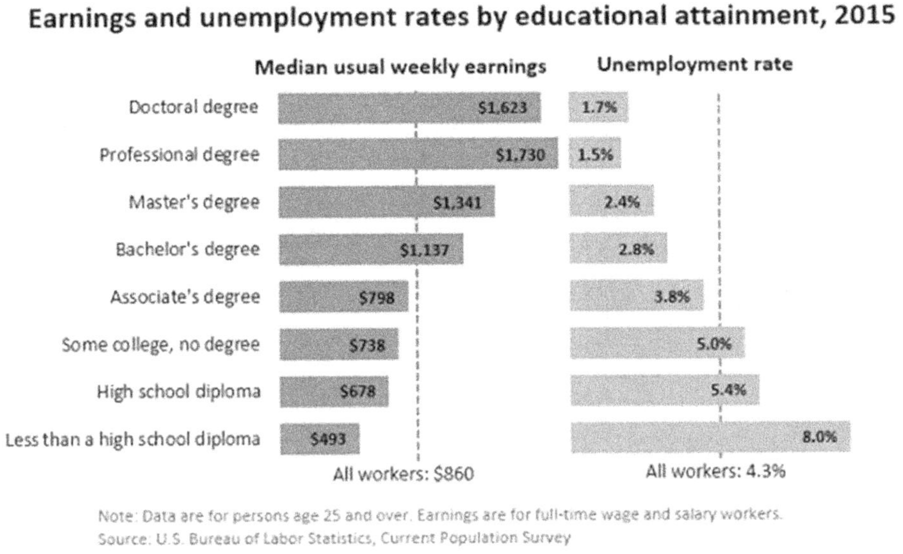

Fig. 7.1 Earnings and unemployment rates by educational attainment 2015 (Source: https://www.bls.gov/emp/ep_chart_001.htm)

The problem with school segregation is that they remain separate but unequal. According to the U.S. Department of Education, who collects data from all public schools in the United States, schools in minority communities have larger class sizes, older textbooks, and less technology. There are also less qualified, less experienced teachers and less access to advanced curriculum like *Advanced Placement* courses in poorer minority schools (U.S. Dept. of Ed. 2016). Many sociologists have also noted differences in the physical condition of school in minority, urban schools compared to White suburban schools. The cracked ceilings, peeling paint, and broken furniture in minority schools can act the same way as teacher expectancy – teachers and students alike can easily get the impression that minority schools are less valued.

The result of school segregation is that minorities, especially African-Americans have lower academic achievement in highly segregated schools that contributes to the achievement gap between minorities and White students. The consequences of the achievement gap are considerable. Education plays a major role in determining a person's life chances. Education is tied to higher earnings and better health status over a person's lifetime. As shown in Fig. 7.1, a college graduate earns nearly twice as much as a high school graduate and is only about one-half as likely to experience joblessness. These are major economic advantages that accumulate over a lifetime.

Education also has health implications. The chart below provides estimates of the number of life years remaining at age 25. What this chart shows is that a 25 year-old woman who drops out of school is expected to live for another 50 years to age

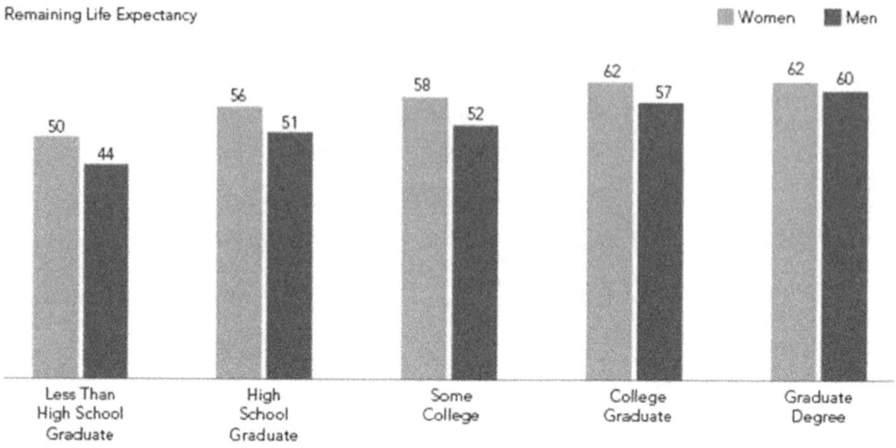

Fig. 7.2 Life expectance at Age 25 by sex and education (Source: Rostron B. L. et al. (2010). Education reporting and classification on death certificates in the United States. *Vital and Health Statistics Series, 2*(151), 1–16. as reported in: http://www.prb.org/Publications/Reports/2013/us-educational-attainment-mortality.aspx)

75. However, if she is a college graduate she will likely live at least another 62 years, to 87 years old. This is a considerable difference. There are many reasons that education contributes to a longer life. More education leads to a better more fulfilling job that is less stressful and pays better. More income also leads to living in a better neighborhood, and having access to resources like quality health care, medications, and higher quality food. All of these things have been shown to increase both the quality and quantity of peoples' lives (Wilkinson and Marmot 2003) (Fig. 7.2).

7.2 Family

When we think of family, we most often picture a nuclear family: a heterosexual married couple with two children who live together in a house. Despite its persistence as a cultural standard, family arrangements also called **kinship** arrangements, are much more diverse. Kinship groups are those connected by blood, marriage, or adoption. Many cultures make a distinction between the family of origin and the family of procreation. The family of origin, also called consanguineous kin, includes family members related by blood (or adoption) including parents, aunts and uncles, cousins. Families of procreation, also called affinal kin, include kinship created through marriage including spouses and their relatives. In many cultures, fictive kin are also recognized. A close family friend may be called a cousin, for example, to recognize their close and kinship-like social ties.

Marriage is fundamental to kinship arrangements. Formally, **marriage** is a legally sanctioned relationship defined by economic cooperation, sexual union, and childrearing. Marriage can take more than one form. Monogamy, the most common form of marriage and by far the dominant form of marriage in the world refers to a marriage between two partners. There are examples, however of polygamy, which is a marriage between more than two people. There are two forms of polygamy: polygyny includes one man and more than one woman and is the most common polygamous form of marriage. Although rare, there are some groups who practice polygyny in the United States including fundamentalist Mormons. Polyandry, a marriage between one woman and more than one man at one time was thought to be very rare. However, a recent anthropological study identified more than 53 different cultural groups around the world that practiced polyandry including Native Americans, native Hawaiians, and a number of other groups throughout Africa and Asia (Starkweather and Hames 2012). Anthropologists believe that the practice of polyandry exists because it provides economic security for women and children in societies with high male death rates.

One may think that marriage is truly an individual choice. However we overlook the many ways in which our choices are constrained by cultural practices, norms and even laws. First, a number of Middle-Eastern and Asian cultures still practice arranged marriages. Second, most marriages are endogamous, or between people with similar social characteristics including race, social class, age, even religion. People tend to be endogamous for a number of reasons. The people we come into contact with, our social groups, are often restricted to where we live, and what schools and churches we attend. Since we tend to interact more with people of the same race and social class, our romantic relationships are often restricted to our familiar social groups. There is also subtle (and not so subtle) family pressure for endogamous romantic relationships. In India, for example, marriage inside one's caste is still important today.

Exogamous marriages, those between people with different characteristics is increasing however. Miscegenation laws used to prevent people of different races from getting married in the United States. In fact, at the turn of the twentieth century, most states legally forbade people of different races to marry. By the 1960s, most states had already overturned the laws, but at least 17 states, mostly in the South, still had laws forbidding interracial marriage. But in 1967, in the now famous Supreme Court decision of Loving vs. the state of Virginia, the court ruled that no state could make a law prohibiting interracial marriage. Since then, the number of interracial marriages has continued to increase. Compared to just a few years ago, when only 1% of marriages were interracial, in 2013 more than 6% of all marriages were interracial (Wang 2015).

After getting married, the decision about where to live is also often culturally determined. A matrilocal residential pattern refers to the expectation that married couples will live with or near the wife's family, while a patrilocal residential pattern means they will live with or near the groom's. These residential patterns often correspond to the patterns of descent. The matrilineal pattern of descent means that property is passed through the maternal line of descent, from mother to daughter. A patrilineal line of descent means that wealth is passed from father to son. China, for example, is strongly patrilineal and patrilocal. Upon marrying, a bride is expected to leave her family and go live with the groom near or with his extended family to help take care of them. This is one of the reasons that sons have been historically favored in China. For a couple, having sons assures that they will be taken care of in old age. Having a daughter means she will leave to go live with her husband's family leaving her parents without support. This preference is so strong that even during a time when the one-child policy was strictly enforced, there were still provisions allowing for a second child if the first was a daughter. The current practice in most contemporary industrialized societies is bilateral descent, in which a married couple recognizes and supports both sets of parents, and property is passed from both sets of parents equally to all their children.

7.2.1 Diversity in Family Forms

As shown in Chap. 5, nearly all Americans say that family is the most important thing in their lives. However, what is considered to be a family is changing. The United States Census Bureau defines families in terms of a household unit. Thus, the definition of a "family household" is one in which at least two people live who are related by birth, marriage, or adoption. This definition excludes a number of households that many of us would define as a family, namely unmarried couples of the same or different sexes living together in long-term relationships. Prior to 2014 same-sex marriages were not recognized in official statistics on family households. However, since that time the census bureau counts all married couples whether gay/lesbian or straight.

Despite the persistence of cultural norms defining married heterosexual couples with children as the "traditional" American family, this is not the dominant type of household in the U.S. As shown in Fig. 7.3, approximately 67% of American households in 2012 could be classified as families. These households include either a married couple with children (20% of the total) or without children (30%). One in five households include single parents living with children and/or other relatives (18%). This means that the "traditional family" makes up only 20% of households, and only about 30% of families. According to the Census Bureau about 1% of US households are same sex couples (married or living together). Although this may not seem like a lot, there has been a substantial increase from 581,000 households in 2010 to more than 850,000 households in 2015, an increase of nearly 50% since 2010.

Stephanie Coontz, in her groundbreaking book "The Way We Never Were" closely examines the short-lived "traditional" American family of the 1950s. She identifies a number of myths associated with traditional families. Among these is the belief that all traditional families were harmonious and stable until the unbridled individualism and feminism of the 1960s and 1970s caused their demise. In fact, perceived stability was often a result of male domination and control. It wasn't until the 1970s that many states began to ban child and spousal abuse. Another myth is that the male breadwinner model, where the woman stays at home, has always been

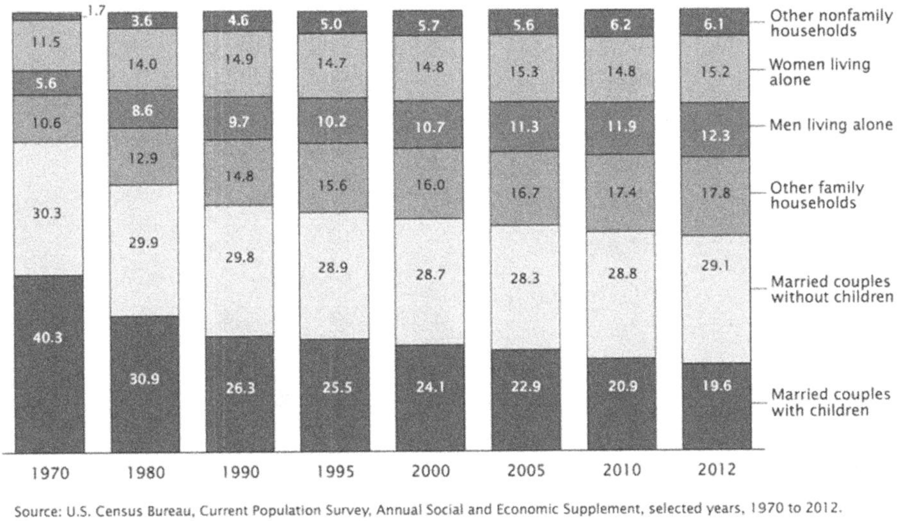

Fig. 7.3 Distribution of household types in the United States 1970–2012

the traditional model. In fact the "traditional" model was that of a wife working hard alongside her husband and her children on a family farm or business. From the 1920s through the 1950s what we now think of as the traditional male breadwinner family emerged, but was no longer the dominant form by the 1970s. She also points out that that many women have had to work to make ends meet in working class families, including in the 1950s.

Since the 1950s, among the most significant changes in American families has been the steep decline in two-parent households, and the equally steep increase in one-parent households. As Fig. 7.4 shows, in the 1960s, nearly 90% of children were living with two parents. That has now declined to about 69%, and the percentage of children residing in single-parent households has increased nearly 3 times, from 9 to 26%. The increase is a result of both divorce and births to single women. Another big change is the percentage of women who remain childless. The percentage of women with a college degree who remain childless by age 40 is nearly 20%. Of women who do have children, they are also having far fewer children. The percentage of women who have given birth who have only 1 or 2 children has nearly doubled from 35 to 63%, while the number of women with 4 or more children has declined from 40 to 14% (Livingston 2015). There are many reasons for shrinking family sizes including increased educational attainment and labor force participation, improvements in contraception, and increased likelihood of remaining single.

There are significant race and class differences among single families. For example, the majority of African American children live in families with a single parent (54%), usually a mother. Similarly, among children born to women lacking a high school diploma nearly half (46%) live in single-parent families. Sociologists have identified economic and racial discrimination as the primary cause of increased

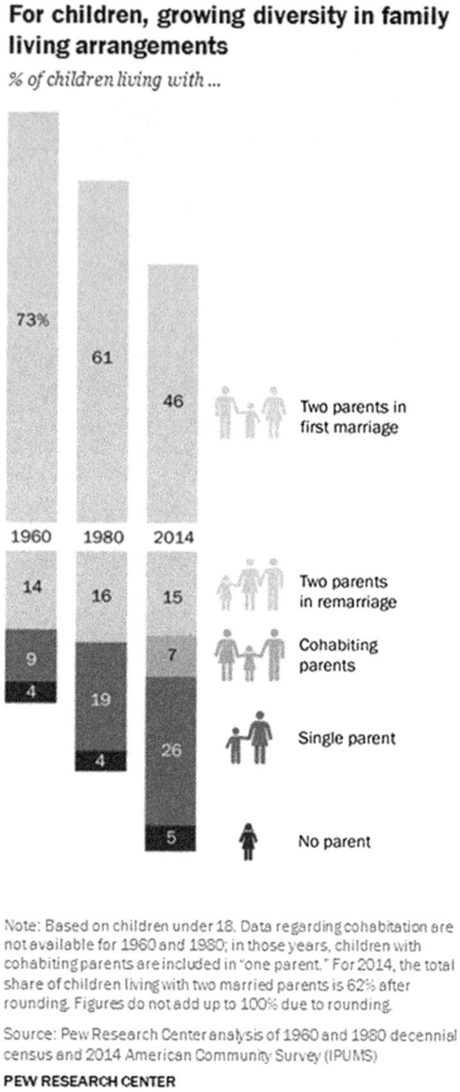

Fig. 7.4 Family diversity in the United States

single-parent households. William Julius Wilson (1987) traced economic and social changes through the middle-of the twentieth century and described how family changes can be traced to the decline in stable manufacturing jobs available to black men in inner cities along with racial discrimination in employment and the criminal justice system. These forces contributed to a decline in the number of young black men who had stable and living wage employment. In fact, as he points out, there were only 50 "marriageable" Black men for every 100 Black women by the end of the twentieth century.

7.2.2 Marriage and Divorce

As shown in Fig. 7.3, the share of American households that consist of married couples have declined dramatically from 70% of households to only 50%, and more than 30% of all children are being raised by a single or cohabiting parents. Does this mean that Americans are abandoning marriage? Not exactly, but there are a number of important social changes that have contributed to the decline in the numbers of married people in the U.S.

First, social norms have changed, and there is now less pressure than ever before to get married. It's more socially acceptable to be a single parent, or cohabiting couple than it was in the past. Sex outside of marriage is no longer considered a social taboo but is viewed as acceptable by at least 60% of Americans (Taylor 2010). Since living together, having sex outside of marriage, and even having children outside of marriage have become more acceptable, more people are delaying marriage or foregoing it all together. In 2010, nearly half of all 25–35 year-olds were not married. That is a dramatic increase from the 1960s when only about 12% were not married.

Second, there are significant economic changes that have affected family life. Women used to be more dependent on men to secure a strong financial future. However, over the past several decades, the pay gap has closed considerably and now women earn about 93% as much as men. Men's wages have also fallen over the past several decades. This is especially true for African American men. Both changes in the availability of good jobs, and racial discrimination have negatively affected African American Men's earning potential. Based on these economic changes, women are not as financially dependent on men as they used to be.

One factor that does not explain the recent decline in marriage is divorce. Although there are still more divorces than there were 50 years ago, the divorce rate has actually been declining since 1980, and so it doesn't explain the more recent decline in married couples. In 1980, the divorce rate in the U.S. was at its highest point ever, just over 5 divorces per 1000 individuals, and it's much lower now at 3.2 divorces per 1000 individuals (CDC 2017). Another way to understand the impact of divorce is by the percentage of marriages ending in divorce. This too has changed significantly. The often quoted statistic that 50% of marriages end in divorce is not true today. Although estimates vary, current estimates suggest that 70% of marriages begun in 1990s have made their 15th anniversary, and people who are married since 2000 are divorcing at even lower rates. It's expected that if current trends continue, only about 35% of marriages will end in divorce. The likelihood of divorce is very different depending on income and education. Only 30% of college graduates are divorced by age 46, compared to 50% of those with only a high school diploma (Aughinbaugh et al. 2013).

7.2.3 *Violence in the Family*

Because families are very private, it's difficult to know how much child abuse, elder abuse, or spousal abuse (also called Intimate Partner Violence or IPV) occurs. Crime statistics underestimate the prevalence of IPV because it is often not reported to the police. Victim surveys are likely better, but may also underreport as victims may feel uncomfortable reporting to a stranger as part of a phone survey. Despite reporting problems, the best estimates still likely come from victim surveys. The National Intimate Partner and Sexual Violence Survey (Breiding et al. 2014) a survey of more than 16,000 adults both men and women reports the lifetime and past-year estimates of sexual, physical, and psychological violence experienced by women and men.

Lifetime estimates suggest that about 10% of women and 2% of men report being raped by an intimate partner and 16% of women and 8% of men report being coerced into unwanted sexual contact. Sexual violence is more often perpetrated by men, and more likely to be perpretrated by a partner, or acquaintance. The National Crime Victimization Survey reports that 78% of sexual assaults were perpetrated by a family member, partner or acquaintance (Planty et al. 2013). Physicial violence was reported by 33% of women and 28% of men, but those liftetime estimates include all forms of violence from a push or shove, to stabbing or shooting. Estimates of severe violence include hitting with a fist or more severe violence and was reported by 24% of women and 14% of men. According to the National Crime Victimization Survey, the incidence of IPV declined over the past two decades, in 1993 5/1000 of women reported abuse now less than 1.5/1000 do. Psychological violence ranges from severe threats of violence, to belittling comments and is equally likely among men and women as 48% of women and 49% of men report experiencing psychological abuse in their relationships at some point in their life.

Sexual, physical, and psychological abuse among intimate partners has significant health impacts. Women who experience abuse are significantly more likely to report depression, anxiety, and suicide attempts. They are also signficantly more likely to use healthcare. Despite high rates of medical care use, at a cost in the billions of dollars, health care providers rarely identify abuse or refer victims to needed social services. In order to help identify and treat victims of IPV, the Agency for HealthCare Research and Quality has developed a toolkit, provided at the end of this chapter, for health care providers to better understand the warning signs and address IPV in medical care settings.

Child abuse is a significant social problem that affects a large number of children in the U.S. The Center for Disease Control (2014) reports that there were over three million referrals, involving 700,000 children who were reported to child protective services. Most were for neglect (78%) but many involved sexual (9%) or physical abuse (9%). These are official reports and likely underestimate the amount of child abuse that occurs since so much abuse goes unreported. According to survey data, as many as 25% of children are maltreated. Athough child abuse has been declining over the past several decades, it remains a signicant social problem.

Even though child abuse occurs among all races and social classes, child abuse is primarily a disease of poverty. Virtually all of the most significant risk factors for child abuse involve social inequality and poverty. These predictors include low family income, unemployment, lack of education, living in a low income neighborhood, stress, and substance abuse. A child living in poverty is five times more likely to be abused than their higher income counterparts (Sedlak et al. 2010).

Just as with IPV, victims of child abuse face significant lifetime health problems. They are at significantly increased risk of imparied cognitive and social development, which also cause long term problems with educational and occupational success. Child abuse also contributes to depression, anxiety, suicide, and drug and alcohol abuse along with an increased risk of heart and lung disease. Since children who experience abuse are significantly more likely to come into contact with the health care system, health care providers have a significant part to play in the detection, intervention, and treatment of abuse. The U.S. Department of Health and Human Services provides a comprehensive set of resources for health care professionals which is available at the end of this chapter.

While both IPV and Child Abuse are declining in the U.S., elder abuse is on the rise along with the increase in the elderly population. As many as 10% of adults over the age of 60 are victims of abuse (Lachs and Pillemer 2015). Because aging adults are often dependent on others to meet their physical needs, elder abuse, like child abuse, includes physical neglect, along with physical and emotional abuse. Many elders also experience financial abuse, when caregivers steal money, or take other resources without consent. Just as with child abuse most elders are abused by their families members. A number of factors also make the reporting and detection of elder abuse difficult. Signs of physical abuse included bruises and broken bones. Signs of emotional abuse include depression and withdrawal of social activities, and signs of neglect include bedsores, poor hygene, and unexplained weightloss. Unfortunately, physical injuries and signs of emotional abuse can also be explained by normal medical issues arising from aging or disease process. Financial abuse can be very hard to detect as well since many seniors are dependent on family members to manage their finances. As with other forms of abuse, elder abuse often goes unreported by healthcare professionals, despite the fact that elders have a great deal of contact with the health care system. It's important for health care providers to learn how to properly assess and intervene in elder abuse (Ahmad et al. 2002).

7.3 Religion

Religion is a social institution that exists in some form in virtually all societies. Its ubiquity is owed, perhaps, to the natural human desire to answer life's big questions like, "why are we here?" and, "what is the meaning of life?" Because the institution of religion is ubiquitous and takes on many forms around the world, it can be difficult to define. In the Elementary Forms of Religious Life (1912) Emile Durkheim defines **religion** as *a unified system of beliefs and practices…which unite into one* *single moral community called a Church, all those who adhere to them.*" Inherent in his definition of religion then, is not just what religion is, a system of beliefs and practices, but what religion does, which is to unite people into a community.

From a functionalist viewpoint (see Chap. 1), religion is universal because it serves a number of important social functions. All religions have group practices or rituals that serve to bring people together on a regular basis in order to create and maintain social cohesion, or connection, among members of a society. It also provides cultural transmission of values and norms from generation to generation as an agent of socialization. Through transmission and maintenance of social norms and values, religion maintains social control and conformity. It also acts to confer legitimacy to the ruling elites. Kings have historically been enthroned through a religious ceremony. In fact, even in the modern U.S., the President is sworn in on a bible and is expected to attend a prayer breakfast soon after taking office. The definition of religion, though, does not include belief in a god, or gods. Theism refers to a religion in which adherents believe in a god or gods. But not all religions are theistic. Buddhism, one of the most widely practiced religions worldwide, for example, has no such deity that created or controls humans. Rather, human fate is determined by the laws of karma as determined by individuals' own actions.

From a conflict perspective, religion serves to support social inequality in a number of ways. One way is by legitimizing political elites who have a stake in maintaining the status quo. Inequality is maintained because the political elites, when ordained by God, will not be challenged by the oppressed who are taught to believe their fate is part of God's will. Karl Marx, in fact, referred to religion as the opiate of the masses because of this. Another important critique of religion is that it supports patriarchy. Christianity and Islam are by their very nature, patriarchal. Religions teach that men are in charge of women, and women should serve men because that is God's will. Thus, religion legitimizes male domination in a patriarchal society. This is changing in modern times, though, as many churches now include women as leaders.

Although there are literally thousands of religions worldwide, there are relatively few major religions that have large numbers of adherents. A study of more than 230 countries worldwide revealed that Christianity and Islam are by far the most widely practiced (Hackett et al. 2012). As Fig. 7.5 shows, more than 50% of the world population identifies with one of those two religions. However, within each of the major religions there are a number of different denominations or subsets of the major religion. For example, within the Christian religion there are Catholics, Protestants, and a number of Orthodox denominations. Even though each of the Christian religions shares a common deity, there are still differences in values, beliefs and norms and rituals that also make them very distinct.

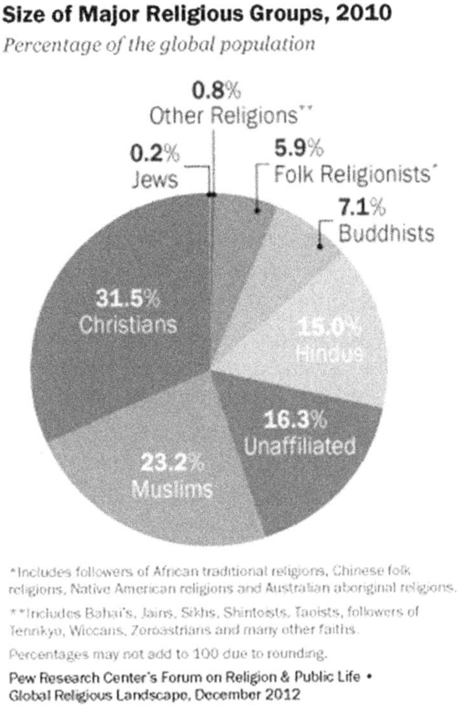

Fig. 7.5 World religions

7.3.1 Types of Religious Organizations

Sociologists often distinguish between different types of religious organizations including a church, a denomination, and sect, and a cult. A **church** is a formal religious organization, often large and bureaucratic with hierarchical leadership. In many countries around the world, the church is formally recognized by the government as a state church. The Church of England (Anglican), the Churches of Norway and Sweden (Lutheran) are examples. Until 1984, when Italy formally separated the Italian government and the Catholic Church, Catholicism was the state religion of Italy. Catholic education was a compulsory part of public education, divorce was against the law, and 90% of Italians were baptized Catholics. The Catholic Church also has a hierarchical and bureaucratic leadership structure from the Pope to local priests.

Many other countries, like France and the United States, have no official state religion, instead there is strict separation between church and state. In these countries, there are many different recognized churches, or denominations. **Denominations** are independent churches, each with its own unique religious doctrine, rituals, and practices. Many denominations, however, also share a common religion. Consider Christianity, there are many different denominations that share in similar Christian beliefs. In the U.S. the Catholic Church, Protestants, Baptists, Methodists, and Presbyterians are all considered different Christian denominations.

These denominations all share a broader common religion but have separated over time because of differences in religious beliefs and practice. The second largest religion in the world, Islam, also includes a number of denominations including Sunni and Shiite that share a common religious tradition but are still separated by beliefs and practices. In practice, the terms "church" and "denomination" are often used interchangeably.

Many recognized denominations were, at one time, sects. A **sect** is a religious organization comprised of a group of people who separate from an established church. Since sects are by definition newly established, they lack the formal bureaucratic structure, resources, and hierarchy of the established churches from which they came. A number of denominations including the Mormon Church, Presbyterians, and Methodists began as sects but grew in size and resources over time to be the well-established denominations they are today.

Cults are religious groups that reject the cultural values of society and form a religious counterculture (see Chap. 5). Like sects, they lack formal organization and bureaucratic structure. Cults most often owe their existence to a charismatic leader and are often short-lived. Doomsday cults often disappear as a result of their end-of-times orientation. The famous Heaven's Gate cult in California was led by Marshall Applewhite, who convinced 39 of his followers to commit suicide in 1997 by drinking poison. Applewhite convinced his followers that the earth was in jeopardy, and to save themselves they needed to drink the poison in order to board a spacecraft sent by God. Other cults run afoul of the law and end when leaders are arrested or killed by law enforcement. David Koresh and many of his Branch Davidian followers were killed in Waco, Texas, in 1993, during a raid by the Federal Bureau of Alcohol, Tobacco, and Firearms. The Davidians were raided as part of an investigation for illegal weapons possession and child abuse. While many cults are short-lived, other cults survive and grow into denominations. The early Christians and Mormons were once considered cults, however, they eventually developed like any other sect, into mainstream churches.

What does it mean to be religious? Sociologists have often grappled with this question. The term **religiosity** is used to describe how important religion is to an individual or group of people. Sociologists measure religiosity along a number of dimensions. One of the ways religiosity is measured is by simply asking people the question: "How important is religion in your life?" Another dimension of religiosity is behavior. Weekly church attendance, for example, is one of the most commonly used measures of religiosity. Finally, another common measure is whether or how often a person prays.

As Table 7.2, shows, at least 80% of Americans say they believe in God. By that measure, then, you would say the majority of Americans are religious. However, if you measure religiosity by church attendance, the answer might be "not very". Fewer than 1/3 of young adults report attending church at least weekly, and in most age groups except the oldest, fewer than 40% do. Religiosity in America is changing as well. Each successive generation, from the Silent Generation to the youngest Millennials, report being less likely to pray or attend church services, less likely to believe in God, and less likely to report that religion is very important in their lives.

Table 7.2 Religious beliefs and attitudes by generation

In many ways, younger Americans are less religious than older Americans

% of U.S. adults who say…

	Silent generation (born 1928–1945)	Baby boomers (born 1946–1964)	Generation X (born 1965–1960)	Older millennials (born 1931–1969)	Younger millennials (born 1990–1996)
Religious behaviors					
They pray daily	67	61	56	46	39
They attend services at least weekly	51	38	34	27	28
Religious beliefs					
They believe in God	92	92	89	84	80
With absolute certainty	71	69	64	54	50
They believe in heaven	75	74	72	67	68
They believe scripture is word of God	69	64	61	50	52
They believe in hell	57	59	59	55	56
Religion's importance					
Religion is very important in their lives	67	59	53	44	38

Source: 2014 Religious Landscape Study, conducted June 4-Sept 30, 5014
PEW RESEARCH CENTER

7.3.2 Religion and Social Change

Religion has been a major force of social change. As Max Weber suggested in *The Protestant Ethic and the Spirit of Capitalism* the religious values of Protestants in the nineteenth century was a driving force behind the development of industrial capitalism. As Weber noted, the Calvinists believed in hard work, self-denial, and frugality. They also believed in investing and accumulating wealth. In fact, the amassing of wealth was seen as a sign of divine blessing. Compared to other religions, including Catholicism that Weber examined, the Calvinists also embraced social change and technological advances in a way other religions did not. Thus, their religious values and attitudes formed the basis for the kind of technological change and accumulation of wealth necessary to usher in the industrial revolution.

There has always been tension between science and religion. Since both are designed to answer questions of meaning in human life. When Copernicus proposed the heliocentric theory in the sixteenth century his book was banned by the Catholic Church, and Galileo was jailed as a result of his own scientific inquiry into the heliocentric theory. This tension between science and religion was addressed by both Durkheim and Weber in their seminal sociological works on religion. And both argued that eventually science, knowledge and rationality would overcome religion as the dominant cultural force in humanity's search for meaning. **Modernization**, as it relates to religion in society, refers to the process by which science and knowledge are increasingly looked to for answers, rather than religion. In the twenty-first century, as debates about climate change, evolution, and the origins of the earth continue, the ongoing tension between science and religion remains evident. It is also clear that given the strong and continuing opposition to scientific findings in each of these categories, religion is still a strong cultural force in America.

Despite the persistence of religion, there is little doubt that much of world is becoming increasingly secular. **Secularization** refers to the declining importance of religion in society. There are a number of different indicators of secularization. Figure 7.5 shows that the third largest group in the world is the unaffiliated. In the U.S., church membership has been declining for decades, and the fastest growing religious group is the unaffiliated who now comprise 22% of Americans. Church attendance is down dramatically as well. Compared to previous generations, the younger millennials are significantly less likely to attend church, or say that religion is important in their life. This doesn't mean that religion is not important anymore. More than three-quarters of Americans still identify with a religion, and most of this group (70%) indicate they are Christian. Religion is still important to be sure, but there is also definitive evidence of secularization in the U.S. Church attendance has declined even more in Europe. In the U.S., 36% of adults report weekly church attendance. In Europe, church attendance is much lower: 3% in Denmark, 5% in Sweden and Finland, 10–15% in France and Germany, and 21% in England. Even in Roman Catholic Italy only 31% report church attendance (Manchin 2004).

Another facet of secularization is the growth of civil religion. **Civil religion**, an idea tracing back to the philosopher Rousseau, refers to the religious deference people have for their nation. Many Americans believe that the United States is more than just a nation, that it is a source of moral virtue in the world and that there is a sacred quality to citizenship. Durkheim defined religion in terms of spiritual beliefs and practices. In fact there are many parallels between religious beliefs and rituals and those commonly found in contemporary civic life. The U.S. Flag is treated as sacred, and there are many rules about how it can be touched and displayed. For many Americans the Flag is the Christian cross, the national anthem is the lord's prayer, the constitution is the bible, and the 4th of July is a religious holiday. To remind ourselves of the importance of our common civil religion, we carry out rituals like the pledge of allegiance, and singing the national anthem before sporting events.

Along with the trend of secularization, there is a parallel trend of growing fundamentalism. There are now more than 62 million Evangelical Protestants in 2014, up nearly 2.5 million from 2007. Along with the religiously unaffiliated, they are the only growing religious group in the U.S. **Fundamentalism** refers to religious groups that believe in maintaining traditional religious beliefs and practices. These include a literal interpretation of religious texts, rejection of religious pluralism, and the enforcement of religious principles by the government. In the U.S., fundamentalist religion is associated political views that oppose abortion, gay rights, and environmentalism (Pew Research Center 2015).

There are strong connections between religion, health, and health care. Oman and Thoresen (2002) reviewed a large number of studies and identified a number of ways that religion has been shown to improve health and longevity. Religious participation can improve social and emotional support known to improve health. It can also lead to improve health behaviors including reduced likelihood of drinking heavily or smoking. It's also likely that religious involvement provides more positive coping mechanisms in times of stress that lead to better cardiovascular health. Scientists are just beginning to learn more about the many ways that spiritual practices including prayer and meditation may improve immune functioning and reduce risks of disease.

The modern hospital developed from charitable religious organizations that cared for the sick and poor. The tradition of church-affiliated hospitals continues to this day, as there are a large number of Catholic and Presbyterian hospital organizations. In fact, among consumer guides that rank hospitals in terms of quality, Catholic and Presbyterian hospitals are often listed among the highest quality hospitals in the nation. Despite the religious name that many hospitals carry, the direct connection between the church and hospital is far less prominent than it used to be. In most cases, the religious affiliation is little more than a name. But it does remind us of the important history of the church in developing hospitals. In nearly all hospitals, whether church affiliated or not, there is a non-denominational chapel where patients and their families can pray or attend religious services. Hospital chaplains, too, are often seen as an important part of the heath care team. Finally, as noted in Chap. 5, many different minority groups have spiritual healers, and those healers are increasingly being integrated into hospital care as a way of incorporating spiritual and physical healing. In short, health care providers increasingly recognize the importance of religion and spirituality for so many of their patients and make attending to both their physical and spiritual needs a priority.

7.4 Government and Politics

Politics may be among the most important institutions that sociologists study because it is the place where the rules and procedures are made that determine the functioning of many other institutions including education, the family, religion and healthcare. It is through **politics** that a society determines the distribution of power, the allocation of resources, and even the goals of a society. The **government** is the formal organization that is responsible for carrying out the political process and enforcing the decisions made. In order to carry out these important functions require that governments exercise power over the social institutions and citizens of a nation.

Max Weber (1921) defined **power** as the ability of individuals or groups to impose their will on others, even in the face of resistance. Power is ubiquitous in society and exists in nearly all, or some would say virtually all, of our social relationships. We are born into power relationships in the family including the power of parents over children, and the power of husbands over wives. In schools, the principal has power over the teachers, and teachers have power over students. The medical profession, too, is extremely hierarchical and full of power relations. Physicians have power over nurses and other medical personnel, as well as patients themselves.

All the examples provided above are examples of **legitimate power** because those who are being controlled consent, and agree with the legitimacy of the power relationship. Sometimes, as in the case of a violent criminal or a military dictatorship, **illegitimate power** is obtained by force and without mutual consent. Most of the power we contend with on a day-to-day basis is legitimate power, and to understand power requires understanding the basis of authority.

Max Weber distinguished between three different types of authority, traditional authority, rational-legal authority, and charismatic authority. **Traditional authority** refers to authority that derives its consent from long standing cultural traditions. That is, a clergyman, a village leader, or even a Chinese emperor or King. Traditional authority is the authority relied upon mostly in pre-industrial societies and made legitimate through cultural traditions, family ties, and often a belief in divine right. It is also the source of authority of many types of traditional healers. As discussed in Chap. 5, spiritual healers are common in many cultures, they have a great deal of power over patients, but their power is the result of cultural beliefs about who they are, not about their formal credentials.

Rational-legal authority derives its legitimate power from laws created and enforced by the government. The power of government officials including elected leaders and those hired to be police, public health professionals, and even teachers are all examples of rational-legal authority. Compared to traditional healers who derive their power from cultural traditions, physicians in the U.S. and other industrialized nations derive their considerable power over other health professionals and patients from laws and regulations enforced by the government. Throughout the 19th and 20th centuries, the health care system was put in place in part through a political process that included standardized and licensed medical education, the licensing of physicians to perform surgery, prescribe medicine, and determine a course of treatment that other health care professionals must follow. In his book titled *The Social Transformation of American Medicine* (1984) Paul Starr traces the social, economic, and political process through which doctors became the powerful group they are today.

Charismatic authority, as the name implies, is authority derived from an individual who possesses a charismatic personality. As described above, the power of a cult leader over their cult stems from charismatic authority. Jesus Christ, Martin Luther King, and Adolf Hitler have all been described by sociologists as charismatic leaders. This is not the same as being a popular leader with rational-legal authority. Charismatic authority is often short lived, or less stable than other forms of authority because the source of power comes from an individual and not a set of cultural or political arrangements. Although short-lived, charismatic authority can also be transformed into rational-legal authority. This occurs when a charismatic leader develops a bureaucratic structure with a hierarchy and governing rules. As described above, the development of the Christian church from a sect into a denomination is an example of the evolution of charismatic to rational-legal authority.

7.4.1 Comparative Political Systems

There are a number of different kinds of political and governmental institutions in existence today. Nearly all are democratic to some degree, but certainly not all. In addition to democracies there are monarchies, and authoritarian and totalitarian states.

A **democracy** is a political system characterized by citizen governance. The central feature of democratic nations is the ability of citizens to vote in free elections. However, free elections are necessary, but not sufficient conditions for democracy. Many so-called democracies have elections, like Mexico, but the elections are run by authoritarian political parties, or many individuals, like women, are excluded from voting. In other cases, there are elections, but the citizens do not have access to a free press, or civil rights that allow them to express their opinions publically or demonstrate. Even in the United States, which is in so many ways a model democracy, there are a number of processes that limit citizens' ability to vote. For example, the formerly incarcerated in many states are not allowed to vote, a rule which disproportionately disenfranchises people of color. Each year, Freedom House a non-profit, nonpartisan organization monitors the state of democracy in 195 countries across the globe. The majority of the nations (45%) in the world are free countries which allow citizens to vote in democratic elections and whose citizens enjoy civil rights protection of their governments. The U.S. and most European countries fall in this category. Another subset (30%), the "partly free" includes countries like Mexico that have elections, but whose citizens' civil rights are not protected. Finally, a number of other countries (25%) around the world like China in which there are neither free elections, nor the exercise of civil rights.

Constitutional Monarchies include countries like England, Denmark, Norway, Sweden and Spain. These political systems are derived from traditional monarchies, in which a divinely ordained monarch commanded absolute power over laws and decision making, and the rule was passed through the same family from generation to generation. With the democratic transformation of these European countries, the monarchies gave way to **constitutional monarchies** in which there are still royal families who participate in government activities in largely ceremonial positions, but the politics of each of these nations are handled by democratically elected parliaments and prime ministers. There are still a few **absolute monarchies** in existence, including Saudi Arabia, Kuwait, and Bahrain. Absolute monarchies, and the name suggests, are government systems in which a royal individual or family have total, or nearly total control over the government institutions and laws of the nation.

Authoritarianism and Totalitarianism: are political systems that do not allow citizens to vote, or freely participate in politics. Authoritarianism refers to a political system, like China's, where an individual or small group of people rule the country, discourage citizens from participating in governance, and severely limit civil liberties including free speech and a free press. Because the Chinese communist party is not freely elected, the state controls all media, and citizens do not have the right to speak out against the government, China would be considered authoritarian. Totalitarianism is even more restrictive. An autocratic ruler or organization maintains control over the population by using illegitimate force, often military force, or heavily militarized police that actively repress citizens. People are imprisoned or killed for speaking out publicly.

7.5 The Economy

The **economic system** is the social institution that ensures the production, distribution, and consumption of all goods and services in a society. As social institutions, economies are embedded in and reflect the unique history and culture of a given society. Rather than a simple mechanistic process through which goods are produced and exchanged, economic systems are fundamentally connected to social systems. As detailed in the preceding section, Weber's work on the link between Protestantism and capitalism described how certain characteristics of the protestant religion led to the development of industrial capitalism. Not only are economic arrangements influenced by culture, but social arrangements and our culture are also influenced by the economy. Consider the many ways in which mass media, an institution driven by the pursuit of profit, has influenced popular culture. Much of our art, music, and film are produced for mass audiences to earn a profit in the free marketplace.

Just as Weber was concerned with the ways in which culture influenced the economy and led to the industrial revolution, Emile Durkheim was interested in the ways the industrial revolution shaped our social arrangements. In *The Division of Labor in Society* (1964, 1893) he described how the industrial revolution shaped the nature of social solidarity. In particular, he noted that with modernization came a more complex **division of labor** in which individuals specialized into narrowly focused occupations. This economic division of labor meant that people had to rely more on each other since no one person or family possessed all the skills necessary to get along. For example, prior to the middle of the nineteenth century, the primary responsibility for medical care resided in the family. There were doctors, but many were not able to make a living as full-time doctors, and so they also had farms of their own or other ways to make ends meet. With the development of modern medicine, the practice of medicine became a more specialized and effective occupation that took years of training. This also meant that doctors worked full time, charged more for their services, and did not have the time for other economic pursuits. A modern society requires a large number of different and specialized occupations that we see today, from bakers and farmers to bankers and construction workers. The basis of social solidarity then shifted from a shared sense of moral values transmitted through religion, which Durkheim called "mechanical solidarity" to true economic interdependence or "organic solidarity."

7.5.1 Comparative Economic Systems

The two major types of economic systems are capitalism and socialism. Since economies are not purely capitalist or socialist, it's best to think about economic systems as existing on a continuum with capitalism on one end, and socialism on the other end. The United States would be closest to the capitalism end of the continuum, and China and Russia would be closer to the socialist end. Most European countries would be somewhere in the middle.

Capitalism is defined by a number of characteristics including private ownership of property and businesses, a "hands-off" government, an individuals' right to pursue profit, free and open market competition, and the freedom of informed consumers to make their own purchasing choices. In capitalist nations, the role of government is limited to running some public institutions like schools, libraries and parks. However, there remains ongoing debate about the extent to which the government in the U.S. should continue its involvement in schools, the delivery of mail, or how large our public park system should be.

The philosophical basis of capitalism is the laissez-faire, or "leave it alone" approach. As Adam Smith believed the key to economic prosperity is to allow the individual pursuit of profit, and that the result would be that goods and services are produced that meet the needs of consumers. The great promise of laissez-faire capitalism is that competition results in high quality and low prices. Informed consumers get to choose between a variety of products that meet their needs, and select the one with the highest quality for the best price. This process ensures that people who sell high quality products will be able to make a living, and for those that buy products they will get good quality at a fair price.

In many ways, capitalism has delivered on its promise. Compared to socialist economies, capitalist economies are highly productive and enjoy greater economic growth. They are also known for having the incentives and the flexibility to continually produce new and innovative goods and services. Because they believe in freedom from government intervention, and free consumer choice, capitalist societies' cultures emphasize the personal freedom of citizens, not just in the marketplace, but also in terms of civil rights and liberties.

On the other hand, there are a number of significant problems with capitalist systems, especially social and economic inequality. As individuals and corporations become successful, they are able to consolidate power and resources and exert control over prices of products and services and wages people receive. Over time, this means a greater share of wealth goes to a relatively small number of individuals, and the gap between rich and poor continues to grow (see Chap. 9). Since the emphasis is on private markets rather than government involvement, people who live on the margins including people with less education and incomes, often lack basic social and economic support and suffer disproportionately compared to those living in socialist nations.

Another shortcoming of capitalism is that is has not been shown to provide high quality health care for a low price. The cost of health care has risen astronomically over the past several years and many people still can't afford to purchase necessary health care services (Bodenheimer and Grumbach 2012). There are a number of reasons that health care does not fit the laissez-faire capitalist approach. First, unlike with other products, people don't choose when or whether they will be sick or injured. This means that health care choices are not usually choices at all, they are imperatives. Second, when buying a car, consumers can shop around, and buy the best quality they can within a particular budget. Health care doesn't work that way. When you have a headache you might need a bottle of ibuprofen for $10 or you might need brain surgery for $200,000. Laissez-faire capitalism also requires that consumers make informed choices. However, because of the specialized nature of health information, people have to rely on information provided by physicians. This means that demand for healthcare is not always based on consumer needs, it's also based on physician referral patterns and consumers don't have the information necessary to judge for themselves whether they are getting what they need. Finally, not all of the costs of health care services are actually paid by the person using them. For example, hospitals are often required to treat patients who come to the emergency room, even if they can't pay. This is like walking into a car dealership, demanding a free car, and being handed a set of keys by the salesman. The difference of course is that no one ever died because they didn't own a car, but every year, thousands of people die because they can't afford healthcare (Wilper et al. 2009).

Socialism is an economic system that is based on public ownership and government control of the production and distribution of goods and services. Whereas capitalism is based on the individual pursuit of profit, socialism is based on working toward the best interest of the community. This means that the focus is on social justice and meeting human needs.

One of the major drawbacks of socialism is that government control often extends into the social realm and citizens lack a number of freedoms that citizens in capitalist nations take for granted. Free speech, freedom of the press, and the freedom of self-determination. Beginning at an early age, many socialist nations track children from an early age into vocational education. Citizens are not always allowed to be what they want to be, but must contribute to the common good of the nation. Citizens in socialist nations are also not allowed to speak out against the government, and state-run media does not allow freedom of the press.

However, may socialist economies including China, Russia, and number of other Asian and Latin American countries, still have inequality, but not to the extent that many capitalist nations, like the U.S., do. Socialist nations do not emphasize keeping wages low in order to boost the profits of private corporations, and are thus more committed to redistribution of wealth that allows all citizens to have a higher standard of living. One of the effects of higher standards of living in socialist nations is the increased health indicators, including lower infant mortality and longer life expectancy (Navarro and Shi 2001).

If capitalist nations are on one end of the continuum, and socialist nations are on the other, a number of Scandinavian and European nations are firmly in the middle. **Democratic Socialism** describes the economic arrangement that includes market capitalism and strong government controls. Countries like Sweden, Norway, Denmark do have government ownership of many industries, but their governments also have strong checks and balances, and there is private ownership of property and business. In many ways, the democratic socialist countries enjoy the best of both worlds. They have very low levels of social inequality, strong national health indicators including very low infant mortality, and very long life expectancy. Much higher than in either purely capitalist or socialist nations. According to convergence theory, capitalist and socialist nations are becoming increasingly similar, as more and more socialist nations like China are slowly allowing market capitalism, and governments in capitalist nations, like the U.S., increase the extent to which the government is involved in regulation and redistribution of wealth.

Key Terms and Definitions

- **Social Structure**: the social arrangements that organize a group or society.
- **Education**: the social institution tasked with transmitting culture and knowledge.
  - **Hidden curriculum**: The informal curriculum in schools where norms, values, attitudes and behaviors are learned.
  - **Teacher expectancy**: The self-fulfilling prophecy in which teachers' expectations of a student or group of students affects their academic achievement.
  - **Educational segregation**: The unequal distribution of minority and White students in schools.
  - **Educational stratification**: The unequal distribution of educational resources in society.
- **Family**: the social institution comprised of kinship arrangements.
  - **Kinship** groups are those connected by blood, marriage, or adoption.
  - **Family of origin**: family members related by blood (or adoption) including parents, aunts and uncles, cousins.
  - Family of procreation: family members through marriage including spouses and their relatives.
  - **Fictive kin**: close family friends referred to using kinship terminology (cousin).
  - **Marriage**: a legally sanctioned relationship defined by economic cooperation, sexual union, and childrearing.

- **Religion**: as a unified system of beliefs and practices which unite all those who adhere to them into one single moral community called a Church.
  - **Religiosity**: the degree to which religion is important to an individual or group of people.
  - **Church**: a formal religious organization, often large and bureaucratic with hierarchical leadership.
  - **Denomination**: independent churches, each with its own unique religious doctrine, rituals, and practices.
  - **Sect**: a religious organization comprised of a group of people who separate from an established church.
  - **Cult**: religious groups that reject the cultural values of society and form a religious counterculture.
  - **Modernization**: the process by which science and knowledge are increasingly looked to for answers, rather than religion.
  - **Secularization**: the declining importance of religion in society.
  - **Fundamentalism**: religious groups that believe in maintaining traditional religious beliefs and practices.
- **Government**: the formal organization that is responsible for carrying out the political process and enforcing the decisions made.
  - **Power**: the ability of individuals or groups to impose their will on others, even in the face of resistance.
  - **Legitimate power**: those who are being controlled consent, and agree with the legitimacy of the power relationship.
  - **Illegitimate power**: power obtained through violence and without mutual consent.
  - **Traditional authority**: refers to authority that derives its consent from long standing cultural traditions.
  - **Rational-legal authority**: derives its legitimate power from laws created and enforced by the government.
  - **Charismatic authority**: authority derived from an individual who possesses a charismatic personality.
  - **Politics**: the social institutions that determine the distribution of power, the allocation of resources, and even the goals of a society.
  - **Democracy**: is a political system characterized by citizen governance.
  - **Constitutional monarchies**: royal families participate in government activities in ceremonial positions, but politics are handled by democratically elected parliaments and prime ministers.
  - **Authoritarianism and Totalitarianism** are political systems that do not allow citizens to vote, or freely participate in politics.
- **Economy**: the social institution that ensures the production, distribution, and consumption of all goods and services in a society.
  - **Capitalism**: The economic system with private ownership of property and businesses, a "hands-off" government, individual rights to pursue profit, free

and open market competition, and the freedom of informed consumers to make their own purchasing choices.

- **Socialism** is an economic system that is based on public ownership and government control of the production and distribution of goods and services.
- **Democratic Socialism** describes the economic arrangement that includes both market capitalism and strong government controls.
- **Division of labor**: Economic system in which individuals specialized into narrowly focused occupations.

Activities

Activity 1: Service Delivery.

Visit the links provided below and examine one or more of the toolkits for working with patients. Describe how this information can be used to improve the delivery of services to patients of varying backgrounds. Consider how your expectations might be different for some groups versus others.

Resources, Links, and Recommended Readings

Recommended Readings

Tatum, Beverly Daniel. 2010. *Why Are All the Black Kids Sitting Together in the Cafeteria?: And Other Conversations about Race*. New York City: Basic Books.

Coontz, Stephanie. 2016. *The Way We Really Are: Coming to Terms with America's Changing Families*. New York City: Basic Books.

Starr, Paul. 2008. *The Social Transformation of American Medicine: The Rise of a Sovereign Profession and the Making of a Vast Industry*. New York City: Basic books.

Bodenheimer, Thomas, and Kevin Grumbach. 2012. *Understanding Health Policy*. McGraw Hill Professional.

Frontline Episode "A Class Divided" Watch Jane Elliott transform her classroom using the power of stereotypes. http://www.pbs.org/wgbh/frontline/film/class-divided/

The Agency for Healthcare Research and Quality Interpersonal Violence prevention toolkit includes a number of resources for identifying and addressing IPV: https://www.ahrq.gov/professionals/prevention-chronic-care/healthier-pregnancy/preventive/partnerviolence.html

United States Department of Health and Human Services Child Welfare Gateway includes resources for identifying, assessing, and intervention: https://www.childwelfare.gov/topics/can/identifying/

The Religious Landscape Survey has collected surveys from more than 35,000 Americans from all 50 states and includes information about religious affiliations, beliefs and practices, and social and political views. The Pew website includes interactive tools to examine data on a wide range of religion topics: http://www.pewforum.org/religious-landscape-study/

Freedom House reports on an annual studies of political rights and civil liberties around the world: https://freedomhouse.org/report-types/freedom-world

Example Study Questions

1. **Define the terms social structure and social institutions.**
2. **How do social institutions influence health outcomes?**

***Example Exam Question:** "Which independent variable would be most appropriate to investigate the impact of primary groups on the outcome measure discussed in the passage?

A. Family structure.
B. Religious affiliation.
C. Occupational status.
D. Population density." (AAMC 2012: 126)

*For more information, visit https://students-residents.aamc.org/applying-medical-school/article/whats-mcat-exam/

References

Ahmad, M., & Lachs, M. S. (2002). Elder abuse and neglect: What physicians can and should do. *Cleveland Clinic Journal of Medicine, 69*(10), 801–808.

Association of American Medical Colleges (AAMC). (2012). *Preview guide for the MCAT 2015 exam* (2nd ed.). www.aamc.org/MCAT2015.

Association of American Medical Colleges (AAMC). (2015). *The official guide to the MCAT exam (MCAT2015)* (4th ed.). Washington, DC: The Association of American Medical Colleges.

Aughinbaugh, A., Robles, O., & Sun, H.. (2013, October). *Marriage and divorce: patterns by gender, race, and educational attainment.* Monthly Labor Review, U.S. Bureau of Labor Statistics, https://doi.org/10.21916/mlr.2013.32

Bodenheimer, T., & Grumbach, K. (2012). *Understanding health policy*. McGraw Hill Professional.

Bowles, S., & Gintis, H. (1976). *Schooling in capitalist America: Educational reform and the contradictions of economic Life*. New York: Basic Books.

Breiding, M. J., Chen, J, & Black., M. C. (2014). *Intimate partner violence in the United States — 2010*. Atlanta: National Center for Injury Prevention and Control, Centers for Disease Control and Prevention. Retrieved from a website at: http://www.futureswithoutviolence.org/userfiles/CDC_Intimate%20Partner%20Violence%20in%20the%20US%20(2010).pdf

CDC. (2017). https://www.cdc.gov/nchs/fastats/marriage-divorce.htm

Eaton, S., & Rivkin, S. (2010). Is desegregation dead? parsing the relationship between achievement and demographics. *Education Next, 10*(4), 50–60.

Friedrich, A., Flunger, B., Nagengast, B., Jonkmann, K., & Trautwein, U. (2015). Pygmalion effects in the classroom: Teacher expectancy effects on students' math achievement. *Contemporary Educational Psychology, 41*, 1–12.

Hackett, C. P., & Grim, B. J. (2012). *The global religious landscape: A report on the size and distribution of the world's major religious groups as of 2010*. Pew Research Center: Pew Forum on Religion & Public Life.

Kerkhoven, A. H., Russo, P., Land-Zandstra, A. M., Saxena, A., & Rodenburg, F. J. (2016). Gender stereotypes in science education resources: A visual content analysis. *PloS One, 11*(11), e0165037. doi:10.1371/journal.pone.0165037.

Lachs, M., & Pillemer, K. A. (2015). Elder abuse. *New England Journal of Medicine, 373*, 1947–1956. doi:10.1056/NEJMra1404688.

Livingston, G. (2015). Childlessness falls, family size grows among highly educated women. Washington, DC: Pew Research Center. *Distributed in any form without written permission from the publisher: American Society on Aging, 575*, 94105-2869.

Manchin, R. (2004). *Religion in Europe: Trust not filling in the pews*. Gallup.com.

Navarro, V., & Shi, L. (2001). The political context of social inequalities and health. *Social Science & Medicine, 52*(3), 481–491.

Oman, D., & Thoresen, C. E. (2002). Does religion cause health?': Differing interpretations and diverse meanings. *Journal of Health Psychology, 7*(4), 365–380.

Orfield, G., & Lee, C. (2006). *Racial transformation and the changing nature of segregation*. Cambridge: The Civil Rights Project at Harvard University.

Pew Research Center. (2015). http://www.pewforum.org/religious-landscape-study/

Planty, M. G., Langton, L., Krebs, C., Berzofsky, M., & Smiley-McDonald, H. (2013). *Female victims of sexual violence, 1994–2010*. Retrieved from a website at: https://www.bjs.gov/content/pub/pdf/fvsv9410.pdf

Rosenthal, R., & Jacobson, L. (1968). Pygmalion in the classroom. *The Urban Review, 3*, 16–20.

Sedlak, A. J., Mettenburg, J., Basena, M., Petta, I., McPherson, K., Greene, A., & Spencer, L. (2010). *Fourth national incidence study of child abuse and neglect (NIS–4): Report to congress*. Washington, DC: U.S. Department of Health and Human Services, Administration for Children and Families.

Starkweather, K. E., & Hames, R. (2012). A survey of nonclassical polyandry. *Human Nature, 23*(2), 149–172.

Taylor, P. (2010). *The decline of marriage and rise of new families*. Pew Research Center.

U.S. Department of Education. (2016). *2013–2014 civil rights data collection: A first look*. Retrieved from https://www2.ed.gov/about/offices/list/ocr/docs/2013-14-first-look.pdf

Wang, W. (2015). Interracial marriage: Who is 'Marrying Out'? *Pew Research Center*. Retrieved from a website at: http://www.pewresearch.org/fact-tank/2015/06/12/interracial-marriage-who-is-marrying-out/

Weber, M. (1921). Economy and society (Vol I, II 1978., ed. and trans. G. Roth & C. W. Mills).

Wilkinson, R., & Marmot, M. (2003). *Social determinants of health: The solid facts* (2nd ed.). Copenhagen: World Health Organization.

Wilper, A. P., Woolhandler, S., Lasser, K. E., McCormick, D., Bor, D. H., & Himmelstein, D. U. (2009). Health insurance and mortality in US adults. *American Journal of Public Health, 99*(12), 2289–2295.

Wilson, W. J. (1987). *The truly disadvantaged*. Chicago: University of Chicago.

Chapter 8
Demographic Structure and Processes

Objectives

- Develop a basic understanding of population dynamics and structures
  - Understand the size and composition of various groups
- Define and discuss major demographic processes: fertility, mortality, and migration
- Consider major shifts related to globalization and urbanization
- Understand how patients' backgrounds contribute to their perceptions of disease, health care, and treatments

Foundational Concept 9
"*Cultural and social differences influence well-being...*

Societal structure, culture and demographic factors influence peoples' health and well-being. Knowledge about basic sociological frameworks, social structures, social institutions, culture and demographic characteristics of societies is important, as is the ability to understand how they shape peoples' lives and their daily interactions" (AAMC 2012: 109).

Category 9B focuses on the demographic characteristics and processes that define a society.

8.1 Demographic Patterns and Their Implications for Health

Racial and ethnic minorities are among the six priority populations, identified by the Agency for Healthcare Research and Quality (AHRQ), for which improvements in chronic conditions, health care access and quality are needed (https://www.ahrq.gov/research/findings/nhqrdr/chartbooks/intro.html). Other groups with priority

G. Garcia-Alexander et al., *Social Foundations of Behavior for the Health Sciences*,
DOI 10.1007/978-3-319-64950-4_8

designations include those with lower socio-economic status (income and education), those in rural locales, children and older adults, sexual and gender minorities (MOGII; for a full list of terminology and definitions see the *Resources* section), and individuals with special needs, disabilities, or multiple chronic conditions (MCC). These demographic characteristics are an important way in which we understand and track the health and wellbeing of various populations. The demographic context of a society provides fundamental knowledge of the basic size, composition, and distribution of various groups within a society. It can further provide us with expectations, or projections, related to the growth and movement of various groups. Those who study population compile highly valuable knowledge of various trends and rates. For example, in the U.S., we formally track births and how they vary by region, race, immigration status, and so on. We further track deaths and their causes along with an entire of series of necessary statistics. This information is vital to needs assessments, resource allocation, and planning for the appropriate care of various groups within society.

In addition, demography provides us with the necessary tools to understand how the relative size of certain groups will change over time (and thus warrant additional investments or specialized attention). For example, racial and ethnic minorities currently comprise 36% of the total population of the U.S., but they are projected to represent half the U.S. population by 2050 (U.S. Census 2012). Racial and ethnic disparities in health outcomes are well-documented, though their sources are less well-understood. Thus, greater investments in research oriented toward understanding the source of disparities will be vital as will investments in solutions that have been shown to improve the health of racial and ethnic minorities. Additionally, developing competence in providing culturally sensitive care will be paramount (Box 8.1).

Box 8.1 Healthy People 2020 Social Determinants of Health Goals
Healthy People 2020 provides a full description of the latest goals and how we need to understand the broad picture to improve health http://www.healthypeople.gov/2020/topics-objectives/topic/social-determinants-of-health

8.2 Demographic Patterns and Structure of the United States

Formally, **demography** is the scientific study of the current state and changes over time in the size, composition, and distribution of populations. Demography is considered a separate discipline in many other countries, but in the United States it is often considered a sub-field of sociology. Demographers track and study the nature of human populations with respect to a number of key structures. The most basic source of demographic information is a census, or count of the population. In the United States, the first census was taken in 1790 and continues today. One can easily access a current count of the population by visiting the U.S. and world population clock (see Resource links at the end of the chapter), which at the time of this writing indicates that the U.S. population is 324,079,993 million people and the world population was 7.34 billion. Information collected by the census is used not only to determine the size and distribution of the population, but to determine things like the crime rate in an area, how to allocate resources such as road expansion/improvement, how many schools are needed for children in the area, and more. This information is also used in the private sector to determine where to locate businesses and to understand the characteristics of the populations in the area. Another important source of demographic information is **vital statistics,** or registration data. These are records of population events including live births, deaths, and marriages, which are compiled continuously using birth, death, and marriage certificate data.

One of the key functions of demography is to understand the composition of populations with respect to certain factors. Demographic structures and characteristics include:

- Age
- Sex/Gender
- Race and Ethnicity
- Immigration Status
- Family Structure/Household Composition (includes sexual orientation)

Age and **sex** are among the most important characteristics in demography, and are actually referred to as "the demographic variables" (Bogue 1969: 147). Age and sex structures of a population have an important impact on the demographic processes of fertility, mortality, and migration. Formally, **age** is defined as a person's age (in years) at their last birthday, and is an ascribed (unchangeable) characteristic. **Sex** is defined as a person's biological sex, i.e. male or female. Sex is, for the most part, an unchanging characteristic which remains the same as that observed at birth. This is in contrast to the more sociological term, **gender**, which refers to the socially constructed aspects and patterns attached to a person's biological sex. As an example, sociologists might investigate gender-based differences in hiring practices. Generally, demographers rely on the term sex to discuss differences in various demographic processes.

Nearly every demographic process varies by age. For example, marriage patterns are heavily dependent on age. Thus, as individuals pass through different stages in life they are more or less likely to experience various events, marriages, migrations, deaths, etc. In addition, the age distribution of a society is equally important. Accordingly, populations that have a higher proportion of young people will differ dramatically from those that have a relatively larger share of older members. An important tool used to understand the age (and sex) distribution of a society is the population pyramid, which illustrates different surviving cohorts of persons of each sex (Poston and Bouvier 2010). The shape of a pyramid indicates how young or old a population is as a whole. As shown in Fig. 8.1, a young population is illustrated by the Democratic Republic of Congo. Young populations have a wide base and narrow toward the top, thus indicating that the birth rate is high (typical of developing

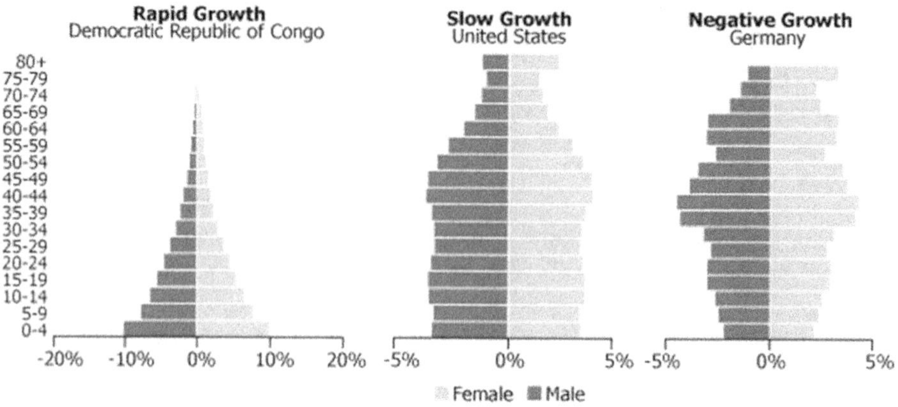

Fig. 8.1 Three patterns of population change (Source: Population Reference Bureau. United Nations, World Population Prospects, The 2006 Revision)

countries) and there are fewer people in the older age groups. A slow growth population is illustrated by the United States. Here' it observed that the shape of the pyramid is more rectangular. This is common in developed countries that have declining fertility and mortality rates. This also reflects a somewhat aging population since the larger bars toward the top mean more people are in the older age groups. One can also observe the bulge of the Baby Boom Generation (they are between the ages of 40–59 in this image). Some countries have actually started to experience zero growth or declining population size as fertility rates continue to decline below replacement levels. Several countries in Europe (including Germany, shown below) are in a situation of population decline and are considered aging populations. Thus, an inverted pyramid reflects a scenario in which death rates exceed birth rates.

Similar to age, the demographic processes are heavily impacted by sex. More specifically, the number of males to females in a society will have measureable effects on everything from marriage patterns, to employment patterns, to women's participation in politics. Sex further impacts mortality, with females experiencing lower death rates at every age and longer life expectancy compared to males. The *sex ratio at birth* (SRB) is a commonly used measure to understand how many males relative to females exist in a society. A balanced SRB is 105 (since males are slightly more likely to die in infancy); meaning 105 males for every 100 females. Thus, by the time a cohort reaches sexual maturity, the number has balanced out. In the United States, we have maintained a stable sex ratio at birth of 105 for many decades. However, several countries have enacted policies that have altered the SRB. For example, in China, the one-child policy, in effect since 1979, limited the number of children families could have to one, and there was a great deal of son preference. This has resulted in a great many excess male births relative to females and an imbalanced ratio as high as 120 (meaning 120 males for every 100 females) in 2000. Concerns ranging from a lack of marriageable females, the spread of sexually transmitted infections (due to the use of sex workers and movement of young men in search of work), and an unprecedented level of lifetime bachelors, among others have arisen. As of October 2015, China did away with the one-child policy in an attempt to deal with population decline and an aging population.

Migration status is another highly important concept to demographers as it reflects one of the three key processes of population change (described in detail below in *Basic Demographic Processes*). Formally, migration refers to the movement of individuals from one location to another, also referred to as **geographic mobility**. We further distinguish between **internal migration**, which is a change of permanent residence within a country; and **international migration**, which is movement between countries. Internal migration is the primary means through which population redistribution within a country occurs (Bogue 1969; Poston and Frisbie 2005). In the United States, we have no restrictions on the internal movement of people, and we keep track the movement of citizens with tools like the Current Population Survey and American Community Survey. We are a mobile population in comparison to many countries with anywhere between 10–20% of the population moving in a given year (Ihrke et al. 2011). But, most people live in the state in which they were born (Ren 2011). The most commonly cited reason for moving is "employment-related reasons," and rates of mobility are highest in those between the ages of 18–29. Following the Great Recession in 2008, demographers witnessed major slowdowns in migration flows. In essence, people were stuck due to a lack of jobs. However, rates seem to be returning to normal and places like the South and West are experiencing some of the highest ever rates of **in-migration** (Frey 2013); meaning they are receiving a great deal of migrants from other states. Figure 8.2 indicates recent national patterns in movement, and indicates those areas of the country that have experienced losses and gains.

The remaining characteristics are not formally considered demographic characteristics, though the social aspects of each have measurable effects on societies as a whole. Race and ethnicity are socially constructed concepts, but we differentiate groups on the basis of both (see Chap. 5 for more detailed information). Formally, race is classified by the U.S. Census, and the 2010 race categories included: White, Black or African American, American Indian or Alaska Native, Asian, Native Hawaiian or Pacific Islander, and Some Other Race (includes all others and multiracial). Data on race have been collected since the first decennial census in 1790. **Ethnicity** refers to Hispanic or Latino and is defined as a person of Cuban, Mexican, Puerto Rican, South or Central American, or other Spanish culture or origin regardless of race (Census 2012). In terms of population distribution, the U.S. is a diverse nation. In 2010, Hispanics made up 16% of the total population, and that reflected a fair amount of growth since 2000 (13%). White alone (non-Hispanic) represented the largest race group at 72% of the total population. Black alone accounted for 13% of the total population in 2010. Less than 1% (0.9) of Americans reported their race as American Indian/Alaska Native or Native Hawaiian/Pacific Islander at 0.9% and 0.2%, respectively. Finally, Asians accounted for 5% of the total population, and the remaining 6% of those reporting a single race reported "some other race" (Humes et al. 2011). The geographic distribution of minority groups also varies. For example, the Western region of the country had a minority population of 33.9 million

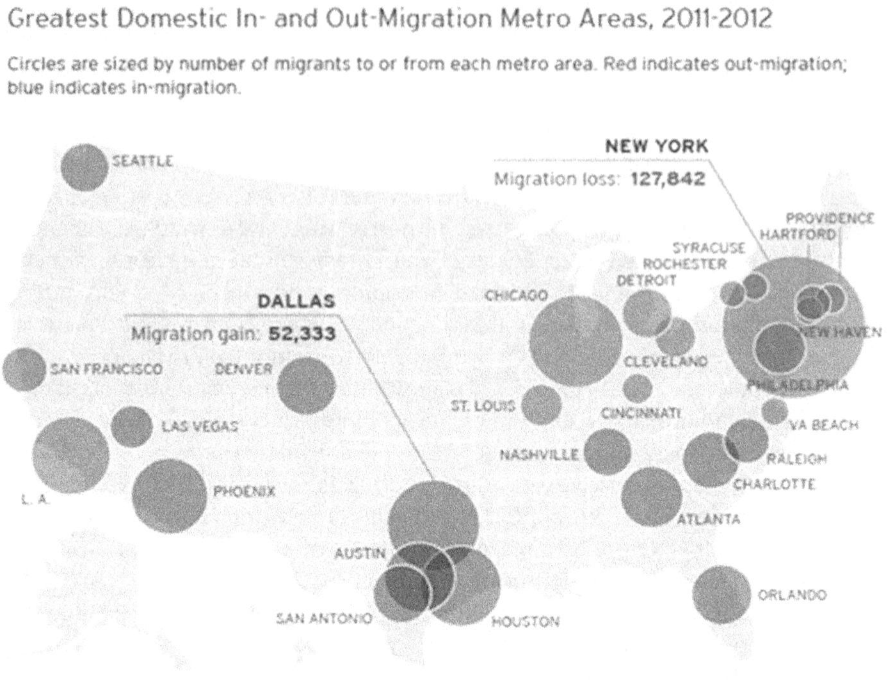

Fig. 8.2 State to state migration patterns (Source: Brookings Institution, State of Metropolitan America, 2013)

(47%) in 2010. Comparatively, the minority population was 40% in the South, 31% in the Northeast, and 22% in the Midwest. In addition, several states have now become "majority-minority" population states, meaning their minority populations were greater than 50%. These include: California, the District of Columbia, Hawaii, New Mexico, and Texas (Humes et al. 2011).

A subfield of demography, known as family demography is devoted to the study of the formation of romantic unions, trends in fertility, changing gender relations, and changes in household size and composition. The definition of family is highly variable from place to place, but the married couple is generally at the center of the family (Waite 2005). In the U.S., household and living arrangements have changed dramatically over time, and there is no real predominant form. This has been in large part due to major changes in patterns of fertility and mortality. Briefly, we have now reached a stage in our demographic transition (discussed below) which is associated with very low birth and death rates, so our families are naturally smaller with fewer children. Changes are also due to declines in marriage (people marry later, cohabit more, and divorce more) and increases in the number of single-parent households. Accordingly, the share of households that were married with children under age 18 decreased from 40% in 1970 to 20% in 2012 (Vespa et al. 2013). In addition, the share of never married individuals has reached its highest point, and nearly 1 in 5 adults over the age of 25 has never married.

An issue of further interest is the rise of alternative family structures, which include gay and lesbian partnerships and cohabiting couples. Indeed, the Census is in the process of improving the quality of estimates of same-sex couples as 37 states now recognize same-sex marriages (Lewis, Bates, and Streeter 2015). A notable change in policy came as a result of the 2013 Supreme Court ruling that the Defense of Marriage Act (DOMA), which was used to bar same-sex couple from receiving federal benefits, was unconstitutional. Still, challenges remain in providing accurate estimates and data on same sex couples. In fact, the first count of same-sex married couples from decennial census came from the 2010 census. Estimates indicate a national total of 902,000 couples (Cohn 2011). Cohabitation has also become an increasingly common structure and refers to a romantic co-residential union. In the United States, this often precedes marriage and either transitions into marriage or is dissolved within a few years (Waite 2005). Increases in cohabiting households have been observed with approximately 7.8 million unmarried partner households in 2012. In comparison, 61 million married partner households were counted in the same time period. Overall, recent general trends in American households suggest smaller family sizes, fewer married couple households, and more people living alone (Vespa et al. 2013).

8.3 The Changing Nature of Society

As my mentor Dudley L. Poston, Jr. commonly used to say, "Demography is destiny!" This phrase refers to the idea that changes to the population structure and distribution produce effects that cannot be controlled and will be felt for generations. In order to fully understand American society, one needs to consider its changing nature and recent demographic shifts. Thus, population dynamics refers to societal level changes in the demographic structure. These often occur in response to some large-scale event. For example, a major shift in the age distribution of society began in the 1950s as a result of a post-war surge in the economy. This led to dramatic increases in the birthrate, which in turn produced what we now refer to as the "Baby Boom" Generation. This cohort, or generation, of individuals refers to anyone born in the years 1946–1964 and is quite large compared to other groups (see Fig. 8.3). As they are reaching retirement age, there are a whole series of considerations with respect to their collective strain on the economic (social security) system, health care (Medicare) system, and social services, i.e. providing care for such a large group of people (see Box 8.2: Further Thought for more info). Formally, in demography a cohort is any group of individuals who experience some major event simultaneously. Thus, there are migration cohorts, birth cohorts, marriage cohorts, and so on.

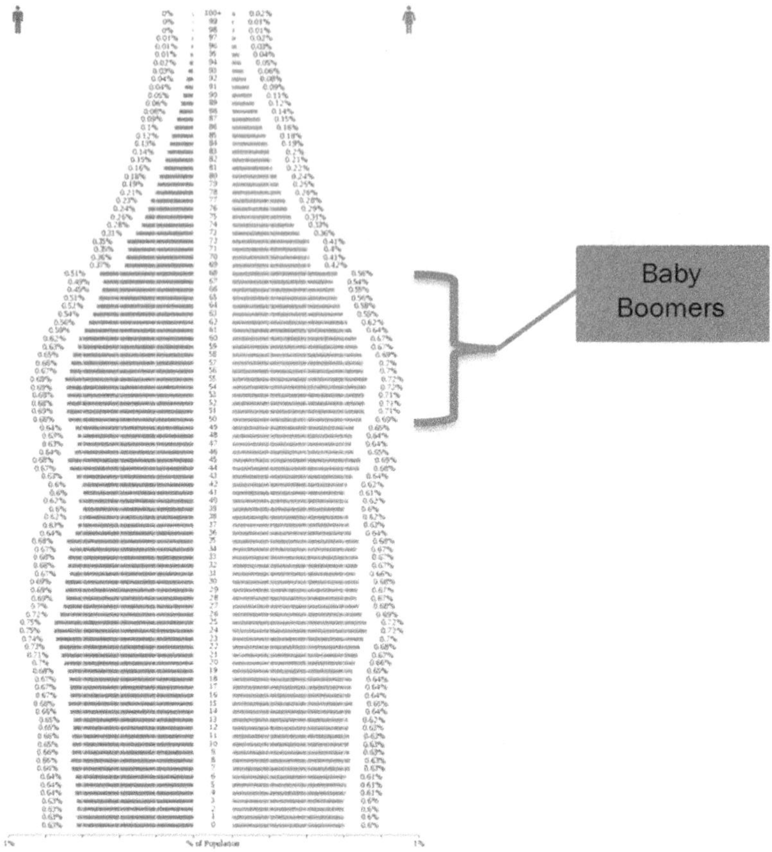

Fig. 8.3 U.S. population, by age and sex, 2015 (Source: U.S. Census Bureau)

Box 8.2: Further Thought: Aging Baby Boomers and Their Health Needs

Demographers and other researchers share concerns over a lack of preparation with respect to the diverse needs of an aging baby boom population. This is the largest age cohort, and they are living longer than those in previous generations. Thus, it is projected that the number of individuals needing nursing home care will increase from 1.3 million in 2010 to 2.3 million in 2030 (Mather et al. 2016). Generally speaking, this cohort has better economic security and levels of education than generations in the past. However, some concerns have arisen over rising obesity in this group, and longer life expectancies means more individuals will live with chronic conditions such as diabetes and high blood pressure. These concerns will be of importance to health professionals and caregivers alike as the nation continues to try address the needs of this large and diverse group.

8.4 Basic Demographic Processes

8.4.1 *Fertility*

Population change or dynamics is organized around the three basic demographic processes of fertility, mortality, and migration. Formally, fertility refers to child-bearing, or the actual production of children. Fertility has a profound impact on the structure of a population and is a major component of population change. Demographers use measures such as the total fertility rate (TFR) to understand fertility patterns in a given population. This particular measure represents the average number of children born to a woman in her lifetime. The 2014 TFR in the U.S. is 1.9, which is down from nearly 2.5 in 1970. Typically, declining fertility is a feature of economic development. Thus, more developed societies have much lower rates of fertility than less developed ones. In 1956, the famous demographers, Kingsley Davis and Judith Blake, wrote about the factors that predict whether a woman of reproductive age will have a child. They referred to these factors as the proximate determinants of fertility, since cultural and economic factors do not directly impact fertility. Instead, they impact a set of variables that directly impact fertility. These proximate determinants include: the proportion of women in a sexual union, the percent of women using contraception, the proportion of infecund (unable to give birth) women, and the level of induced abortion (Bongaarts 1978). Together, these factors explain nearly all the variation in fertility rates in populations. Depending on the context, some factors are more important than others. For example, in the U.S. contraception and abortion are the most important factors in explaining fertility rates.

Declining fertility rates are a common feature of many developed countries. In the U.S., fertility rates remained around 7 children per women until the 1800s. Fertility steadily declined until the 1970s when it reached its lowest point of 1.74 in 1976. This occurred because of widespread contraceptive use, delayed marriage, and abortion (McFalls 2007). The current rate of 1.9 will likely not increase since more and more women are delaying marriage and childbirth. Fertility rates are considered *low* if they are below replacement level; and they are considered *lowest-low* if they are at or below 1.3 (Billari and Kohler 2004). At present, several European (Poland, Romania (1.3), Portugal (1.2)) and Asian (China, Japan, Taiwan (1.2)) countries are experiencing lowest-low fertility, which is thought to be the product of increased labor force participation in women and delayed childbearing. Many are concerned about this issue since it impacts the dependency ratio. This is a measure that indicates how many people there are in working age relative to those in dependent age groups (those younger than 15 and those older than 64). As fertility levels continue to decrease, the ratio of working age individuals shrinks and thus pulls into question how societies will care for a growing elderly population.

8.4.2 *Mortality*

Another major component of population change is mortality, which is the subtraction of people (as opposed to addition via fertility). Death rates provide us with an understanding of the number of people who die in a given year, but they do not provide us with an understanding of well-being of the citizens in a population. A better measure of well-being comes to us in the form of life expectancy. This measure indicates how long an individual can expect to live and allows us to compare various populations/nations. For example, as of 2016, the life expectancy at birth in the U.S. was 76 among men and 81 among men. In comparison, the life expectancy at birth in 49 among men and 52 among women in the Democratic Republic of Congo. At the other end of the spectrum, the country with the highest/best is San Marino at 84 among men and 89 among women (World Population Datasheet 2016). We further see variations in life expectancy within populations on the basis of such characteristics as sex, age, race, and socioeconomic status (SES). For example, SES has consistently been linked to health and mortality outcomes with those at higher levels enjoying successively longer and healthier lives. This finding is referred to as the social gradient in health.

Another indicator of population well-being is the infant mortality rate (IMR). This particular measure reflects how many infant deaths occur per 1000 live births in a given year. In the U.S., we have a remarkably high IMR despite the level of economic development. This is attributable to the level of inequality present among certain groups. Thus, we see very high rates of infant mortality in Black and American Indian women. On the other hand, we observe very low rates of infant mortality in White and Asian women.

8.4.3 *Demographic Transition Theory*

One of the most prominent theoretical perspectives in demography is **Demographic Transition Theory** (Thompson 1929; Notestein 1945), which links fertility and mortality changes to the process of industrialization and urbanization. For most of human history the population was very small. In fact, the population was never greater than 10 million until the seventeenth century when agrarian societies began to develop, and by the 1800s the world population reached 1 billion (McFalls 2007). As societies begin to industrialize, they pass through four stages in the demographic transition. In the first, births and deaths remain quite high, thus the population size remains relatively stable as people have many births, but high death rates negate any rapid population growth. This first stage is referred to as the pre-industrialization stage. As populations achieve economic development, the amount of deaths due to famines and epidemics begin to decrease. Thus, the overall mortality rate declines but the birth rate remains high since it takes a little longer for couples to realize they need fewer children. This is a period of rapid population growth and falling

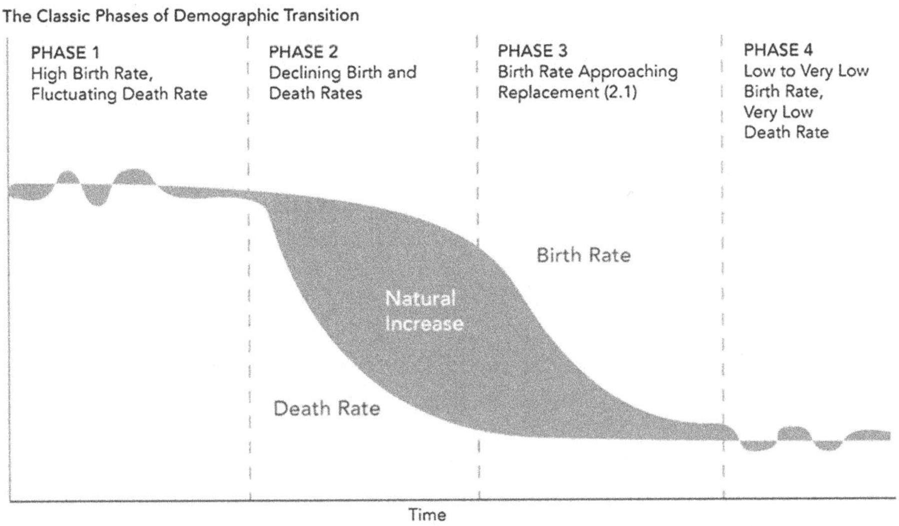

Fig. 8.4 Demographic transition (Source: https://www.newsecuritybeat.org/2011/08/prbs-population-data-sheet-2011-the-demographic-divide/)

mortality rates. As couples realize they need fewer children, they begin to control their fertility, and thus the birth rate drops as well. This third phase is one of falling birth and death rates (decreasing population growth). Finally, birth and death rates "bottom out" and reach a stable low level in which families are small. In Europe this transition occurred over 200 years (between 1800 and 2005) and during this time the population increased by four times. During this same time frame in North America the population was multiplied by 63 (INED 2008). Today, America ranks third in overall population size (behind China and India). Some countries have still not fully achieved their demographic transitions and remain in the second or third phase of the transition (Fig. 8.4).

8.4.4 Migration

A final component of population change is migration. This particular component can result in the addition of (in-migration) or subtraction of (out-migration) people from a population. It also happens to be the least stable of the processes discussed since it is highly sensitive to external events. As mentioned above, demographers have noted a slowdown in internal migration (Frey 2009). In fact, internal migration reached its lowest point since WWII in 2008. However, migration trends seem to have changed yet again as economic recovery has resulted in increased movement to certain locations (see Fig. 8.2).

International migration refers to the movement of people between countries. Formally, the term **immigration** (in-migration) reflects the movement of people into a country to settle; while the term **emigration** (out-migration) refers to the movement of people out of a country. Globally, international migration has increased to 244 million in 2015 from 222 million in 2000. Unlike many other countries, the U.S. allows relatively unrestricted immigration and hosted 47 million immigrants in 2015 (up from 35 million in 2000) (UN 2015a). In fact, the U.S. receives more immigrants than any other country in the world. Migration is highly selective, with the young, educated, and able-bodied most likely to immigrate. Males slightly outnumber females in patterns of immigration, and the median age of global migrants was 39 in 2015 (UN 2015a). Immigration can occur as a result of what are referred to as "push" or "pull" factors. *Push factors* are those that encourage the individual to leave an area and include job loss, major catastrophic events, lack of availability of marriage partners and so on. On the other hand, *pull factors* are those that attract individuals and include such things as job/economic opportunities or better living conditions.

The history of immigration in the U.S. has witnessed some major shifts in the composition of immigrants, which can be thought of in waves. The *First Great Wave* occurred in the period between 1820 and 1880 and was driven primarily by the need to meet labor demands brought on by industrialization. During this time, the U.S. hosted 4 million immigrants (the greatest influx in history) from Britain, Germany, Ireland, China, and Mexico. The *Second Great Wave* occurred between 1880 and through the First World War. During this period, the growth of industry in Great Britain and Germany created labor demands in those countries, thus dampening the stream to the U.S. Meanwhile, unemployment in Southern and Eastern Europe led to a new stream of immigrants from countries including Italy, Russia, Poland, and Greece. Close to 25 million immigrants came to the U.S. during this period. In 1924, the National Origins Quota Act imposed strict sanctions on immigration; in effect massively reducing the flow of immigrants up until the 1960s. This is referred to as the long hiatus in immigration (Massey 1995). Several factors played a role in this hiatus including national origins quotas directed specifically at Southern & Eastern European and Chinese immigrants (fueled by nativist sentiments), the outbreak of a world war, the Great Depression, and increased demand for labor in sending countries following the war.

Finally, the Third Great Wave, also called the *New Regime* (Massey 1995), occurred in the period between 1960 and 2000. Fewer than 10% of the immigrants in this time frame came from Europe. Instead, the majority came from Latin American and Asian countries. Indeed, the majority came from just four countries: Mexico, the Philippines, Vietnam, and El Salvador (Massey 1995). In more recent years, we have seen some additional shifts as fewer immigrants are coming from Mexico. Recent findings actually suggest that more Mexicans are leaving the U.S. than entering. However, this country is still the largest contributor to the U.S. immigrant stock. Other countries that have increased in the number of immigrants to the U.S. are China and India, with both sending 2 million in 2015 (UN 2015a). In consideration of overall population dynamics, only Hispanic and Asian groups have seen considerable growth in their populations between the 2000 and 2010 Censuses, mainly due to higher levels of immigration. Importantly, more than half the growth between 2000 and 2010 was attributable to increases in the Hispanic population (Humes et al. 2011).

In the Health Setting: Generally speaking, the health of foreign-born immigrants is better than that of native-born individuals in the U.S. Accordingly, acculturation (or the adoption of the attitudes, beliefs, and norms of the host culture) is associated with poorer health outcomes. In other words, the health habits of immigrants grow worse in accordance with more time spent in the U.S. For example, increased acculturation has been association with higher rates of cancer and infant mortality (Abraído-Lanza 2006). On the other hand, Hispanics have consistently evidenced relatively favorable mortality outcomes. Thus, an important concept introduced by social demographers is the *Hispanic or epidemiologic paradox* (Markides and Coreil 1986). This is a concept that refers to research findings which suggest that the health and mortality of Hispanics as a group is better than what would be expected given their comparatively lower socioeconomic position. Several explanations have been developed to account for these findings. The first is the *healthy migrant* hypothesis. This argument suggests that selection effects account for the better health of foreign-born Hispanics. In other words, those who are in better health to begin with are the ones who are more likely to migrate. Another explanation is *salmon bias*, or *return migrant effect*, which has been proposed to account for lower mortality rates in this group and argues that foreign-born migrants return to their host countries to die – thus artificially lowering their rates of mortality. A final explanation is the *health behaviors* hypothesis, which suggests that immigrants engage in better health behaviors and have fewer risk factors (they are less likely to smoke, have better diets, and less alcohol consumption). However, as mentioned above, research has also shown that health behaviors worsen with acculturation. Demographers remain unclear on the exact causes of a mortality advantage among Hispanics. For a selection of readings on the paradox see the *Resources* section.

8.5 Ongoing and Projected Shifts in Society

The current world population is 7.3 billion, and the population of the U.S. is 324 million. Demographers project that the world population will reach in 8.5 billion by 2030 and 9.7 billion by 2050 (United Nations 2015). Much of the growth in the world population is expected to occur in nine countries (including the United States which is expected to reach 388 million by 2050) (United Nations 2015).

In the United States, growth comes from two sources (natural increase and migration). First, fertility rates are a bit higher than they are in other developed countries. The U.S. population also continues to grow due to immigration. One of the most noteworthy shifts in the U.S. pertains to its multiracial composition. We are in the midst of dramatic changes to the nature of the American population that include a declining White majority, an increasing minority population, a greater presence of Latin American and Asian immigrants, and more multi-racial marriages (Frey 2013). These shifts are accompanied by intense cultural and generational divides, which have recently manifested in a historically unprecedented level of contention in the political landscape. Younger generations evidence a much higher degree of racial inclusiveness and tolerance, which will be needed given projected demographic trends.

8.5.1 Urbanization

An important trend in population dynamics has been the one toward increased **urbanization**. This refers to the proportion of the population living in urban places (Weeks 2008). At present, more people live in urban areas that in rural ones globally, which is a major reversal of living arrangements observed throughout human history. This trend will continue and it is projected that about two-thirds of the world population will live in urban areas by 2050 (United Nations 2014). Some areas are urbanizing faster than others, however. For example, more than 75% of the populations in North and Latin America and the Caribbean are urban. In comparison, Africa and Asia have larger shares of rural populations (though their urban expansion is occurring faster here than in other regions) (UN 2014). We have also seen a trend toward large and "**megacities**." Indeed, these "mega-cities" (cities with 10million + inhabitants) are expected to continue to grow and will house a large share of the world's population. Today, there are 28 global mega-cities. But, it expected that there will be 41 mega-cities by 2030. These will include: Tokyo, Delhi, Shanghai, Mumbai, and Beijing, among others.

Here in the U.S., we have experienced some redistribution of the population. Certain metropolitan areas have experienced high rates of growth (10% or more per year), while others have declined in population. Some de-concentration of metropolitan areas has also been observed. This is a process whereby people settle the outlying, lightly settled areas surrounding metros, and is known as **suburbanization**. Between 1960 and 2000 the number of suburban dwellers in the U.S. more than doubled from 61.9 million to 124.8 million (Guest and Brown 2006). However, recent data suggests that migration to suburbs has decreased (Frey 2013). We have also seen some urbanization trends and recent findings suggest that there have been gains in large urban cores like San Francisco, Boston, and New York (Frey 2009).

A final concept pertaining to the distribution of the population that has long been examined by demographers is **segregation**. This refers to the physical separation of groups along the lines of social class, race/ethnicity, or other characteristics. In the U.S., segregation on the basis of race has been a persistent feature of the population. Scholars in this area contend that though there has been some decline in Black-White segregation in smaller cities in the South and West; larger metropolitan areas in the Northeast and Midwest that house the majority of Black populations remain highly segregated (Massey 2004). Indeed, the term **hypersegregation** has been developed to describe the experience of segregation along multiple dimensions. From a health standpoint, a great deal of literature has examined the health consequences of residential segregation. Research findings suggest that the conditions produced by segregation, i.e. concentrated poverty, social disorder, and poorer access to educational and economic oopportunities, lead to negative health outcomes (Williams and Collins 2001).

8.5.2 Globalization

Globalization refers to economic, political, and cultural processes that include the rise to dominance of the transnational corporation, the rise of information and service economies, the growth of international organizations, and the spread of global consumption, information, and exchange (Ritzer and Ryan 2010). Countries across the globe vary dramatically in their composition and structure and each face a unique set of challenges. Globally, standards of living have increased, but some countries have experienced worsening conditions and global inequality is increasing. However, increasing globalization will ensure that the challenges of other countries will be felt across the globe. For example, political instability or war in one region of the world may lead to immigration issues in many other regions; air travel and increased mobility may open up the possibility for global public health concerns; increased consumption trends will have a major impact on the planet's resources; and food shortages in regions that produce a large share of the world food supply could have widespread effects. Health concerns have also increased as a product of globalization and urbanization. For example, we have seen the re-emergence infectious diseases thought to be extinct (now antibiotic resistant) made possible by the movement of pathogens across global borders. Urbanization contributes to this process as the vast majority of humans live in urban centers that act as incubators for infectious diseases. Climate change will add to this burden. For additional information on this topic see the *Resources* section.

Global population growth and urbanization bring concerns over scarcity of resources, the potential for the development of urban slums, depopulation in some areas, and a reduced quality of life for future generations. Those with a keen eye will recognize the need for smart policies that consider that consider the role of family planning and immigration policies. Additionally, the need for global sustainable policies with respect to urbanization cannot be overstated. Urban growth offers opportunities to expand access to services and care, but these resources must be distributed evenly. It is also important to avoid excessive centralization and the development of urban slums. Further, environmentally sustainable cities must be developed in order to accommodate the needs of a growing population and preserve Earth's resources.

Key Terms and Definitions

- **Demography** (Content Category 9B): the scientific study of human populations and its processes of change including fertility, mortality, and migration.
- **Vital Statistics**: records of population events including live births, deaths, and marriages, which are compiled continuously using birth, death, and marriage certificate data.
- **Demographic Structures**: population characteristics, such as age and sex, that are used to tabulate the size, composition, and distribution of a human population; also used to track changes in population
- **Demographic Processes**: three main factors or components of change in a population
  - **Fertility**: refers to the actual production of live *births* that occur in a population.
    - **Fecundity**: the ability to produce children
  - **Mortality**: deaths that occur in a population.
  - **Migration**: the movement of people from one geographic area to another to establish a new residence; also referred to as *geographic mobility*
    - **Internal Migration**: a change of permanent residence within a country; may refer to regional or state to state relocation
      - **In-migration**: the residential migration of persons to an area of destination
      - **Out-migration**: the residential migration of persons from an area of origin
    - **International Migration** (Content Category 9B): the movement of individuals from one country to another on a permanent or semi-permanent basis
      - **Immigration**: the movement of people into a country to settle
      - **Emigration**: the movement of people out of a country
      - **Undocumented Migration**: the relocation of individuals into a country within which they have not been granted legal rights to do so; categories of undocumented migrants include visa-overstayers and those who enter illegally
- **Demographic Transition Theory**: a theory that explains the changes fertility and mortality as a result of modernization. The transition occurs in four phases including the pre-industrialization, early industrial/falling mortality, declining fertility and mortality, and incipient decline.
- **Globalization**: increases in economic, political, and social interconnections across the world.

- **Urbanization**: increases in the percent or proportion of the population living in urban, densely-settled areas.
  - **Mega-cities**: (also called megalopolis) a term used to describe very densely populated urban settlements with 10 million or more inhabitants.
  - **Suburbanization**: a shift from higher-density central cities to lower-density areas outside the city limits
  - **Segregation**: the formal and informal separation of one group from another; often on the basis of demographic characteristics including race/ethnicity, gender, or religion.

Activities and Research Examples

Activity 1: American Factfinder.

Use the American FactFinder (or Social Explorer) to examine the area you intend to serve. Alternately, you can choose to examine the place where you grew up. What are its demographic characteristics? What are the health conditions that are prevalent in the area? Consider things such as: which is the largest racial/ethnic group, what is the age structure, what is the overall size of the population, how many physicians per capita are there? Further consider how and why these characteristics may be connected to the presence of various chronic conditions.

Activity 2: Global Trends Quiz.

Test your understanding of the population trends and challenges facing the world. Quiz accessible through from the NOVA "World in the Balance" site: http://www.pbs.org/wgbh/nova/earth/global-trends-quiz.html

Activity 3: Example impacts in the health setting.

From "Think Cultural Health" https://cccm.thinkculturalhealth.hhs.gov/: "Within 50 years, nearly half of the nation's population will be from cultures other than White/non-Hispanic, increasing the provision of medical services to patients of diverse cultures or languages. Cultural and language differences may engender misunderstanding, lack of compliance, or other factors that negatively influence clinical situations." How can these practices be incorporated? Who is needed on staff to ensure such needs are met? Visit the site above to learn about ways to prepare.

Research Example 1. Baby Boomers.

People in the healthcare profession will increasingly need to account for the care of the Baby Boom Generation as they move fully into retirement. Some have suggested that they are in worse condition than previous generations in terms of chronic conditions. In addition, this is an incredibly diverse group with large gaps in health on the basis of race, class, and education. Read the report: Aging in the United States (http://www.prb.org/pdf16/aging-us-population-bulletin.pdf) and consider/discuss the impacts this group will have and plans to meet the needs of this group.

Resources, Links, and Recommended Readings

Recommended Readings on the Epidemiologic/Hispanic Paradox:

Abraído-Lanza, A. F., Dohrenwend, B. P., Ng-Mak, D. S., & Turner, J. B. (1999). The Latino mortality paradox: a test of the "salmon bias" and healthy migrant hypotheses. *American Journal of Public Health, 89*, 1543–1548.

Akresh, I., R., & Frank, R. (2008). Health selection among new immigrants. *American Journal of Public Health, 98*(11), 1–7.

Hummer, R. A., Powers, D. A., Pullum, S. G., Gossman, G. L., & Frisbie, W. P. (2007). Paradox found (again): Infant mortality among the Mexican-Origin population in the United States. *Demography, 44*(3), 441–57.

Markides, K. S., & Coreil, J. (1986). The health of hispanics in the southwestern united states: an epidemiologic paradox. *Public Health Reports, 101*(3), 253–265.

Palloni, A., & Elizabeth Arias. (2004). Paradox lost: Explaining the hispanic adult mortality advantage. *Demography,41*(3), 385–415.

Recommended Readings on the Urbanization/Globalization and Health:

Armelagos, G. J., & Harper, K. N. (2009). Emerging infectious diseases, urbanization, and globalization in the time of global warming. In W. C. Cockerham (Ed.), *The new blackwell companion to medical sociology*, Oxford: Wiley-Blackwell. doi:10.1002/9781444314786.ch13

McMichael, A. J. (2000). The urban environment and health in a world of increasing globalization: Issues for developing countries. *Bulletin of the World Health Organization, 78*, 1117–26.

General Readings:

McFalls, J. A. (2007). *Population: A Lively Introduction* (5th ed.). *Population Bulletin, 62*(1).

U.S. Census Population Clock: http://www.census.gov/popclock/

National Institute of Demography: The National Institute of Demography website contains an informative and useful set of videos and infographics on population growth and change. http://www.ined.fr/en/everything_about_population/videos/

Population Reference Bureau. PRB is an excellent resource that compiles and analyzes complex demographic data. Website provides access to World Population Datasheets, informative videos, articles, reports, lesson plans, and a data finder. www.prb.org

Racial and ethnic minorities http://www.ahrq.gov/research/findings/nhqrdr/nhdr13/chap11.html

United Nations Population Division. Provides demographic estimates and projections for all countries, monitors progress and global health, hosts major population and development conferences. http://www.un.org/en/development/desa/population/about/index.shtml

Example Study Questions

4. **Describe the major findings with respect to the overall health of various racial and ethnic groups. Which groups tend to have the bets outcomes across a number of different diseases and conditions? Conversely, which groups tend to do the worst?**

***Sample portion of passageand example from exam:** "Low birth weight is a risk factor associated with less favorable health and developmental outcomes later in childhood and adolescence. In the United States, low birth weight is disproportionately prevalent among racial and ethnic minority groups and has been linked to specific environmental and social characteristics of neighborhoods.

***Example Exam Question:** Assuming the differences reported in Table 1 are statistically significant, what can be inferred about Latino mothers in the sample?

A. Latinos live in less segregated neighborhoods than do Asian-American mothers.
B. Latinos live in more segregated neighborhoods than do African-American mothers.
C. Latinos are less likely to have low-birthweight infants than are African-American mothers.
D. Latinos are more likely to have low-birthweight infants than are Asian-American mothers." (AAMC 2012: 125)

*For more information, visit https://students-residents.aamc.org/applying-medical-school/article/whats-mcat-exam/

References

Abraído-Lanza, A. F., Armbrister, A. N., Flórez, K. R., & Aguirre, A. N. (2006). Toward a theory-driven model of acculturation in public Health Research. *American Journal of Public Health, 96*(8), 1342–1346.

Association of American Medical Colleges (AAMC). (2012). *Preview guide for the MCAT 2015 exam* (2nd ed.). www.aamc.org/MCAT2015.

Billari, F., & Kohler, H.-P. (2004). Patterns of low and lowest-low fertility in Europe. *Population Studies, 58*(2), 161–176.

Bogue, D. (1969). *Principles of demography*. New York: Wiley.

Bongaarts, J. (1978). A framework for analyzing the proximate determinants of fertility. *Population and Development Review, 4*(1), 105–132. doi:10.2307/1972149.

Cohn, D.'. V. (2011). *How accurate are counts of same-sex couples?* Washington, DC: Pew Research Center.

Frey, W. H. (2009). *The great American migration slowdown: Regional and metropolitan dimensions*. Washington, DC: Brookings Institution.

Frey, W. H. (2013). *Economic improvement nudges U.S. migration to normal*. Washington, DC: Brookings Institution. http://www.brookings.edu/research/opinions/2013/03/15-us-migration-economics-frey.
Guest, A. M., & Brown, S. K. (2006). Population distribution and suburbanization. In In D. L. Poston Jr. & M. Micklin) (Eds.), *Handbook of population*. New York: Springer.
Humes, K. R., Jones, N. A., & Ramirez, R. R. (2011). *Overview of Race and Hispanic Origin: 2010, 2010 Census Briefs*. Washington, DC: U.S. Census Bureau. http://www.census.gov/library/publications/2011/dec/c2010br-02.html.
Ihrke, D. K., Faber, C. S., & Koerber, W. K. (2011). *Geographical mobility: 2008 to 2009, Current population reports, P20–565*. Washington, DC: U.S. Census Bureau.
Institut National D'Etudes Demographiques (INED). (2008). *The demographic transition*. Animation Series: The World Population. Accessed at: https://www.ined.fr/en/everything_about_population/videos/the-demographic-transition/
Lewis, J. M., Bates, N, & Streeter, M. (2015). *Measuring same-sex couples: The what and who of misreporting on relationship and sex*. Social, economic, & housing statistics division working paper, Washington, DC: US Census Bureau.
Massey, D. S. (1995). The new immigration and ethnicity in the United States. *Population and Development Review 21*(3): 631–652. doi:1. Retrieved from http://www.jstor.org.proxy.lib.pdx.edu/stable/2137753 doi:1
Massey, D. S. (2004). Segregation and stratification: A biosocial perspective. *Du Bois Review, 1*(01), 7–25.
Mather, M., Jacobsen, L. A., & Pollard, K. M. (2016). Aging in the United States. *Population Bulletin, 70*(2), 2–3.
McFalls, J. A., Jr. (2007). Population: A lively introduction. *Population Bulletin, 62*(1), 1–31.
Notestein, F. W. (1945). Population: The long view. In *Food for the World* (pp. 36–57). Chicago: University of Chicago Press.
Poston, D. L., Jr., & Bouvier, L. F. (2010). *Population and society: An introduction to demography*. New York: Cambridge University Press.
Poston, D. L., Jr., & Frisbie, P. (2005). Ecological demography. In D. L. Poston Jr. & M. Micklin (Eds.), *Handbook of population* (pp. 601–623). Springer: New York.
Ren, Ping. (2011). *Lifetime mobility in the United States: 2010*. U.S. Census Bureau. https://www.census.gov/library/publications/2011/acs/acsbr10-07.html
Ritzer, G., & Michael Ryan, J. (2010). *The concise encyclopedia of sociology*. Chichester: Wiley-Blackwell.
Thompson, W. S. (1929). Population. *American Journal of Sociology, 34*(6), 959–975.
U.S. Census Bureau. (2012). "*Census Bureau reports National Mover Rate Incraeses after a record low in 2011*." News Release, American Community Survey, Washington, DC. https://www.census.gov/newsroom/releases/archives/mobility_of_the_population/cb12-240.html
United Nations, Department of Economic and Social Affairs, Population Division. (2014). World urbanization prospects: The 2014 revision, highlights (ST/ESA/SER.A/352).
United Nations, Department of Economic and Social Affairs, Population Division. (2015). World population prospects: The 2015 revision, custom data acquired via website.
Vespa, J., Lewis, J. M., & Kreider, R. M. (2013). *America's Families and Living Arrangements: 2012, Current Population Reports, P20–570*. Washington, DC: U.S. Census Bureau. http://www.census.gov/library/publications/2013/demo/p20-570.html.
Waite, L. J. (2005). Marriage and family. In D. L. Poston Jr. & M. Micklin (Eds.), *Handbook of population*. New York, Springer.
Williams, D. R., & Collins, C. (2001). Racial residential segregation: A fundamental cause of racial disparities in health. *Public Health Reports, 116*(5), 404–416.

Chapter 9
Social Inequality and Stratification

Objectives

- Introduce basic concepts and theories of stratification
- Examine the ways in which inequalities are distributed within societies and by social class, gender and race/ethnicity

Foundational Concept 8

Psychological, socio-cultural, and biological factors influence the way we think about ourselves and others.

"Human beings are social by nature. Though the sentiment is simple, the actions and processes underlying and shaping our social interactions are not" (AAMC 2012: 108).

Category 8B (*social thinking*) focuses on the processes that contribute to prejudice and bias (power, prestige, and class).

Category 8C (*social interactions*) focuses on the actions and processes underlying social interactions and discrimination (how power, prestige, and class facilitate discrimination).

Foundational Concept 10

Social stratification and access to resources influence well-being.

Category 10A (*Social inequality*) focuses on a broad understanding of social class, including theories of stratification, social mobility, and poverty.

"Barriers to the access of institutional resources exist for the segment of the population that is disenfranchised, and/or lacks power within a given society" (AAMC 2012: 113).

G. Garcia-Alexander et al., *Social Foundations of Behavior for the Health Sciences*,
DOI 10.1007/978-3-319-64950-4_9

9.1 Social Class

This chapter addresses the mechanisms of how social relations lead to social inequalities observed by social class, race/ethnicity, and gender, which create and shape disparities in health (see Chap. 10 for more detailed discussion on health disparities across various social groups). Although the term **social class** is one of the most frequently used concepts in sociology, there is no clear agreement about how the notion of social class should be defined. Most sociologists use the term to refer to socioeconomic variations in their material prosperity and power, and it often is measured by income, wealth, education, and occupation. Sociologists tend to focus on how there are many layered dimensions to this concept; and it is a product of one's status, which is determined not only by their material wealth, but also by the amount of power we have access to. This is in turn determined by the roles and statuses we occupy. Social class is often used together with the term **stratification**, which is defined as systematic inequalities between groups of people.

Different forms of class systems exist, and sociologists examine how material resources and power are acquired in order to characterize a society. For example, a *caste system* is one in which people are born into their class position and cannot change it by virtue of achievement. Thus, they have access to resources on the basis of their **ascribed status**, i.e. the status they are born with. An example of a society exhibiting a caste system is Hindus in India. Another example is the system of apartheid that was once in place in South Africa. A **meritocracy** refers to a social stratification system based on personal merit, or a person's knowledge, skills and effort. We have no evidence of any complete meritocracies, though our current society values an individual's credentials. Thus, we live in a society in which people are placed in various positions, such as lower-class, middle-class, etc. on the basis of their **achieved status**. The dominant perspective on this situation in our society is that people reside in the category they have earned. Meaning, we believe in the idea that our *achieved statuses* will lead to the ability to secure a position in the category we wish to belong to (as opposed to our *ascribed status*). Some additional detail and varying perspectives on this are provided in the following.

9.1.1 Theories of Stratification

One of the founders of sociology, Karl Marx, contributed a great deal to the study of social class in society. In his seminal work on class, *Das Kapital* (originally published in 1867), he extensively details the social hierarchy and how each of us is placed in it on the basis of our economic position. He thus assigns class to people on the basis of their relationship to the means of production – the means by which people gain a livelihood. According to Marxism, there are the two main classes, the *bourgeoisie* (or capitalists) who own the means of production, and the *proletariat*, or the workers, who do not own the means of production. The proletariat should therefore earn their living by selling their labor to the capitalists. He considers the relationship between classes exploitative in nature – given that the inherent goal of capitalists is to maximize the surplus value while minimizing costs. According to Marx, this exploitative system would ultimately lead to revolution by the working class as they came to recognize their needs in opposition to those who owned the means of production in capitalist societies (i.e. **class consciousness**). Accordingly, this term refers to the development of a sense of shared identity. In comparison, **false consciousness** refers to the state in which classes are unaware of their subordinate position and thus prevented from organizing on the basis of their true interest.

Another founder of sociology, Max Weber extends on Marxism, given that he conceptualizes the distinction between classes as being a product of more than just an economic relationship to the means of production. First, he emphasizes not only the ownership of the means of production, but also other resources, such as skills and credentials to explain where class divisions derive from. Thus, he believed that a person's place in society was based on a combination of legal, political, and cultural criteria, in addition to their economic position. Additionally, while class is an objective measure (determined by whether one owns means of production or not), he also used "status," a subjective evaluation of social differences, to refer to the social honor or prestige that people assign to various roles and positions in a society. In its simplest form, **status** refers to the position that a person occupies in the social order. Weber thought of classes as groups of people who shared similar *life chances*. Lastly, Weber recognized another dimension, **power**, which refers to one's ability to enact change, control resources, command decisions. This concept is central to his perspective on social stratification and is formally defined as the ability, "[of men] to realise their own will in a communal action even against resistance of others who are participating in the action (Weber 1922, recited from Coser 1977: 230). He considered power to be of primary importance, and both class and status were seen as dimensions of that.

9.2 Social Stratification in Contemporary Societies

9.2.1 Social Class Position

One's social class, often identified in terms of education, income, wealth, power, and occupational prestige, is critical in influencing a person's life chances, including their health status. As mentioned above, our stratification system is one in which we are able to exert a certain degree of **social mobility**. This refers to the idea that we are able to change our position through our achievements (more details on this concept are provided below). In the United States, we observe both upward and downward mobility, meaning a person can move up or down in the social ranks. Unfortunately, we have also observed that the opportunities for advancement are diminished for women as well as racial and ethnic minorities.

Generally, the term inequality refers to a system of unequal rewards and opportunities for groups or individuals in a society, and it is a concept that has received much attention in sociology and other disciplines. *Socioeconomic status* (SES) is a commonly used way of identifying someone's position in the social hierarchy. An expanding body of literature has developed that confirms the strong and enduring association between a person's SES and their health. For health professionals, it is especially important to understand this relationship and how it may translate into poorer health outcomes (that should not be assumed to be due to some failing or unwillingness on the part of the individual). Thus, inequality can have direct and indirect impacts on health. In a direct way, inequality can produce differing levels of access to high quality health care and providers. In an indirect way, it can impact health because it may produce differences in the amount of social support a person has access to or the health and safety of the neighborhoods in which they reside.

Income inequality is a term that describes a situation where there are gaps in earnings and earnings potential across various social classes. In terms of global and historical trends, it has been observed that as societies develop, their level of income inequality reduces. But, it seems that income inequality increases in post-industrial societies, a trend that was not predicted by those who saw development as a positive outcome. In the United States, we have observed increasing levels of distance between the upper and lower classes. This inequality has been increasing steadily since the mid-1970s, and has been attributed to low wages, a service economy, increasing female workforce participation, and limited public assistance, among other issues. Formally, **income** refers to earnings from paid work as well as other sources such as investments. Comparatively, **wealth** is the total value of assets that a person owns after deducting debts. Material resources of income and wealth are considered important sources of **power**. Importantly, various ascribed and achieved characteristics influence our earnings potential, power, and ultimate position in the social hierarchy.

Education influences occupation and income, thus leading some people to have greater opportunities in the pursuit of higher education than others. In this way, education, or access to it, can reproduce social and income inequalities. Finally, **occupational prestige** refers to prestige that some occupations offer. For example, white-collar occupations offer higher prestige compared to blue-collar ones.

While there are no universal designations of social class that sociologists all agree on, recent descriptions of the following four categories are useful for understanding broad class differences in the US (Giddens et al. 2016; Proctor et al. 2016; Ritzer and Ryan 2010):

Upper class	The upper class consists of the very wealthiest groups with more than $200 K households income or approximately 5% of all American households
Middle class	The middle class composed of those working in white-collar and lower managerial occupation. Their income ranges between $40K and $200K, roughly including 55% of all households. Because it is such a broad category, the middle class is often further divided in to the upper middle class for those with income from $100K to $200K (almost 20%), and the lower middle class for those whose income is lower than $100K (about 40%).

(continued)

Working class	The working class includes primarily blue-collar workers and the household incomes range from $20K to $40K. This group comprises about 20% of all American households.
Lower Class	The lower class includes some full-time low-wage workers, those who work part-time, or unemployed. Their annual household income is typically lower than $20K. Many people in this group live in poverty without benefits such as medical insurance, disability, or Social Security.

9.2.2 *Racial and Ethnic Inequality*

Ascribed status can have a real and measureable impact on a person's life chances and lead to differential access to education and other resources that directly affect achievement. Racial and ethnic status is an example of such an ascribed status, and is known to directly influence the resources one has access to. Sociologists recognize that there are not any real biological differences that produce these differences – these are social differences that are produced and maintained by the social order (for more information see Chap. 6). This creates differences in educational attainment levels, housing opportunities, the potential for wealth accumulation, neighborhood safety, likelihood of imprisonment, and so on. As an example, the figure below (Fig. 9.1) indicates that although overall increases in the real median

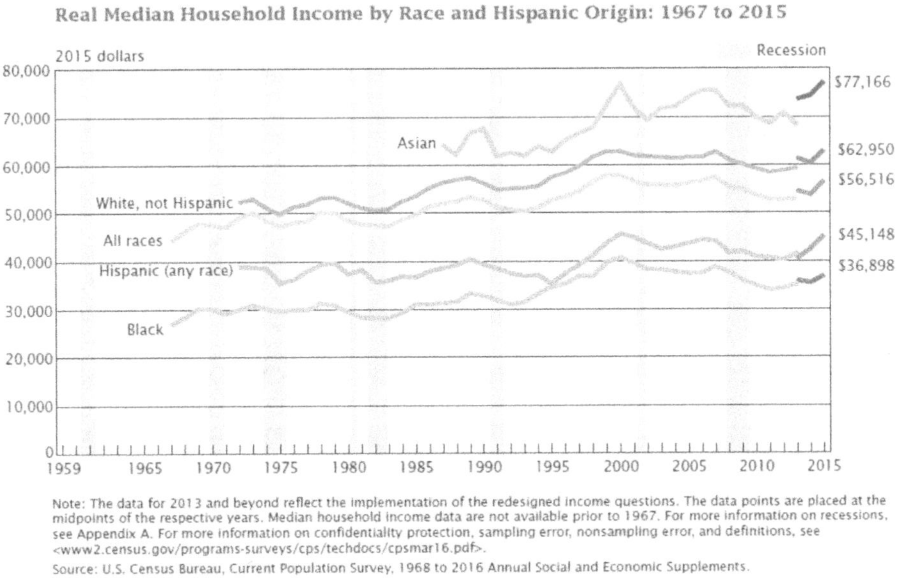

Fig. 9.1 Real median household income by race and hispanic origin: 1967–2015 (Proctor et al. 2016: p. 5)

household income are observed for all race and ethnic groups over the past several decades, substantial income disparities have persisted. Specifically, the real median income for non-Hispanic whites in 2015 was $62,950, compared to a median income of $36,898 among non-Hispanic. The real median household income for Hispanics was higher than that observed among NH Blacks, but it is much lower than the median income for non-Hispanic whites. These differences are largely attributable to variation in the educational attainment of these group members.

9.2.3 *Gender Inequality*

Gender inequality refers to differences in the social status, power, and prestige that women experience in relation to men in a society. Most sociologists agree that a certain level of disadvantage is associated with female status, which translates into differences in the occupational structure, their representation in politics, and the household division of labor. For example, work that is considered women's work has a tendency to be undervalued in our society, and this is reflected in associated earnings and job security for these types of jobs. Some progress has been made in this area, and as seen in the below figure, the gender wage gap has narrowed over time. However, a substantial gap has persisted such that as of 2015, women earn 80% of what men do on average (Fig. 9.2).

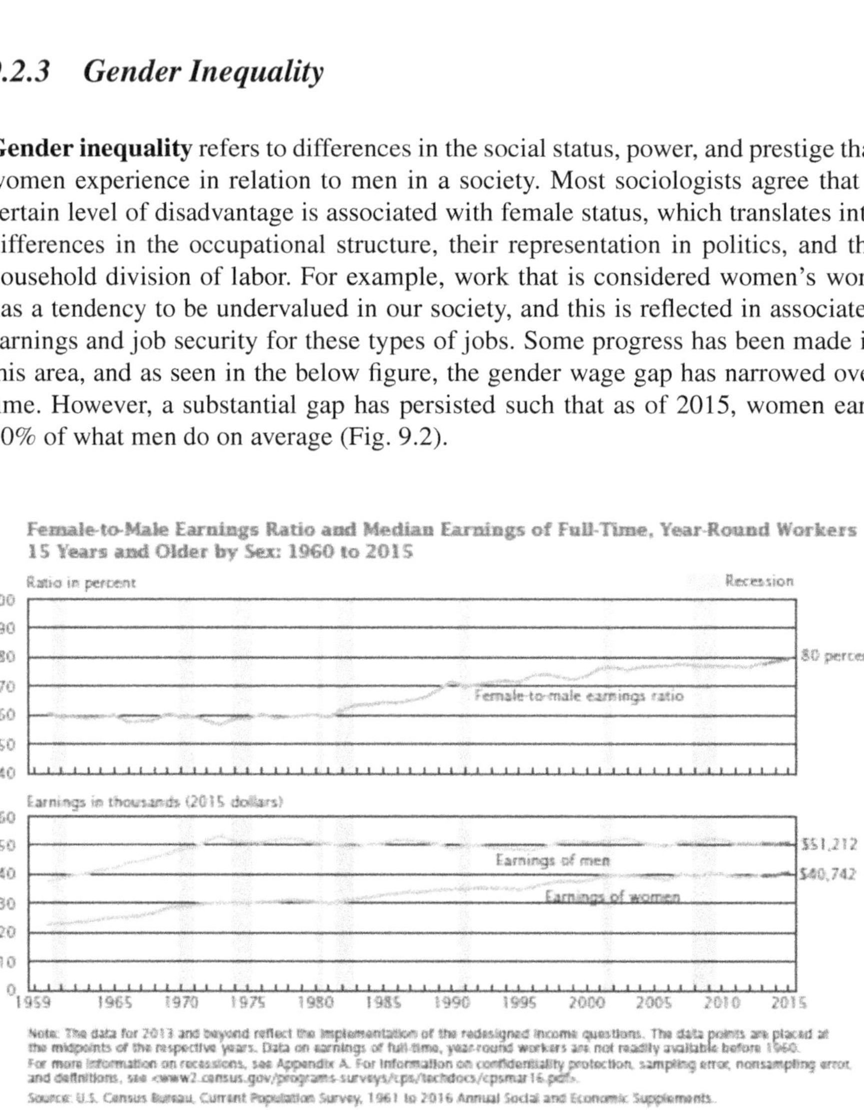

Fig. 9.2 Female-to-male earnings ratio and median earnings of full-time, year-round workers 15 years and older by sex: 1960–2015 (Proctor et al. 2016: p. 10)

What explains gender inequality? Sociologists have provided several insights on *occupational segregation* and *gender discrimination* at work. The first explanation relates to the fact that women tend to work in poorly paid occupations, such as clerks, or secretaries. This brings down their average earnings potential. However, this is changing as educational attainment has increased among women. Thus, greater proportions of women are pursuing more prestigious jobs, such as lawyers or physicians, in recent years. Nonetheless, a high concentration of women in low-status occupations is still observed. For example, over 94% of secretaries are female (US Bureau of Labor Statistics 2015). The second explanation that helps us to understand a persistent gender-based earnings gap is *gender discrimination*. Generally, this concept suggests that women are at a disadvantage in the workplace via institutional and interpersonal discrimination. For example, women working in male-dominated occupations often face a 'glass ceiling', or an upper barrier, that prevents them from getting promoted.

9.2.4 Spatial Inequality

Segregation is the physical and social separation of people by certain categories (Macionis 2014). Although some religious groups, such as the Amish, or subcultures may voluntarily isolate themselves from the larger society, **residential segregation** occurs when majority group members work toward the exclusion of minorities in the housing setting resulting in neighborhoods that are not characterized by a high degree of racial or ethnic diversity. Even after the Brown v. Board of Education of Topeka, in which the Supreme Court overturned a system of segregation (known as Jim Crow Laws, which allowed for "separate but equal" pubic facilities) in public schools, residential segregation continues to persist in the US. Similarly, there exists a high degree of educational segregation between blacks and whites in large metropolitan areas as residential segregation across race and ethnicity persists.

9.2.5 Measures of Segregation

Massey and Denton (1988) provides us with five key dimension of residential segregation that are useful for measuring its presence. These include: *evenness*, *exposure*, *concentration*, *centralization* and *clustering*. First, **evenness** reflects the differential distribution of the population of interest. The most widely used measure of evenness is the dissimilarity index, which measures "the proportion of minority members that would have to change their area of residence to achieve an even distribution, with the number of minority members moving being expressed as a proportion of the number that would have to move under conditions of maximum segregation" (Massey and Denton, p. 284). Values of the dissimilarity index range from 0 (when no minority members would have to move) to 1 (when all minority members would have to move). Second, **exposure** "measures the degree of potential contact or possibility of interaction, between minority and majority group members" (Massey and Denton, p. 287), and the isolation index is commonly used as a measure of this. The third dimension is **concentration**. Using a measure known as the Delta Index, concentration measures "the relative amount of physical space occupied by a minority group in the metropolitan area" (Massey and Denton, p. 289). When minority groups of the same or similar size occupy less space, the area is considered more concentrated and therefore more segregated. Fourth, **centralization** measures "the degree to which a group is spatially located near the center of an urban area" (Massey and Denton, p. 291). The Absolute Centralization Index is often used to measure centralization. Lastly, **clustering**, measured by the Spatial Proximity Index, refers to the extent to which areal units inhabited by minority members adjoin to another, or cluster, in space (Massey and Denton, p. 293) (Figs. 9.3, 9.4, 9.5, 9.6 and 9.7).

To get a better idea of the places with the most and least segregation in the US, several images are shown below (Figs. 9.8 and 9.9). As can be observed, the most racially segregated large metropolitan area in 2000 was Milwaukee-Waukesha, WI (U.S. Census). By contrast, the least segregated large metropolitan area was Orange Country, CA.

9.2.6 Neighborhood Safety and Violence

Residential segregation directly impacts inequality in public schooling. Neighborhoods greatly differ on the basis of the resources and funding they have for schools. As schools are typically funded through local property taxes, children in more affluent neighborhoods receive better educations compared to those living in poorer neighborhoods. For example, the average salary of public school teacher in South Dakota is $39,580 (as of 2012–2013), but it was $75,279 in New York (US Department of Education 2013). Additionally, graduation rates vary across the states. For example, Washington D.C. has a 60% graduation rate, while Iowa has over 90% graduation rates (US Department of Education 2015).

Education is among the most important predictors of economic resources. Similarly, inequalities in public schooling and educational outcomes are impacted by variations in the level of neighborhood safety and violence. Because racial and ethnic minorities are more often concentrated in disadvantaged neighborhood, the areas where racial and ethnicity minorities are predominantly located often exhibit higher levels of crime and violence. As a result, people residing in these areas are more often exposed to higher levels of air pollution, noise, unemployment, fewer grocery stores, and insufficient access to and availability of health care facilities.

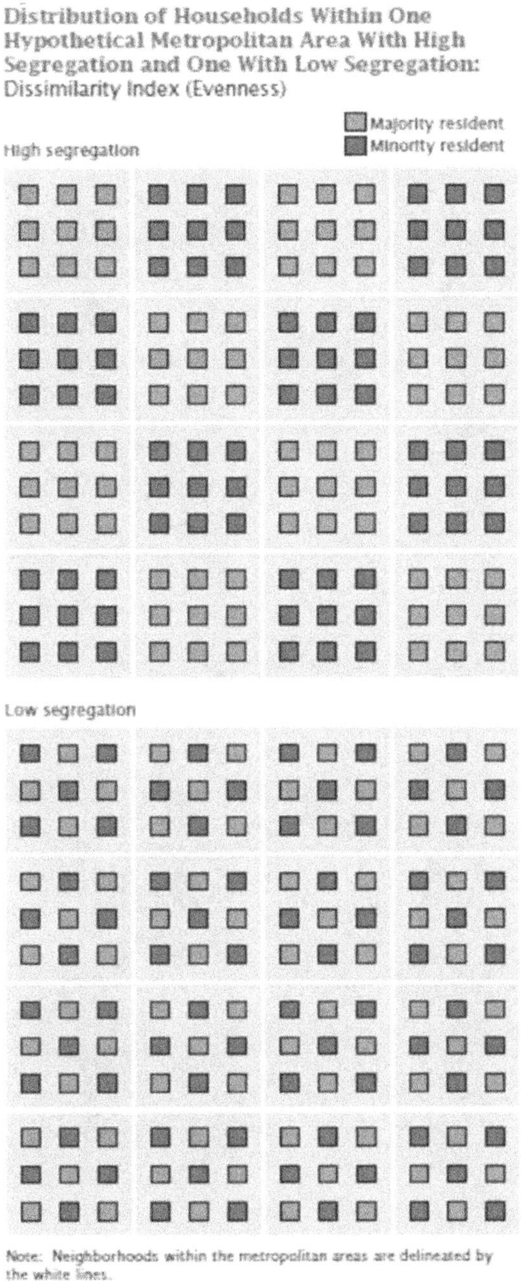

Fig. 9.3 Illustrations of segregation measures – dissimilarity index (Iceland et al. 2002: 9)

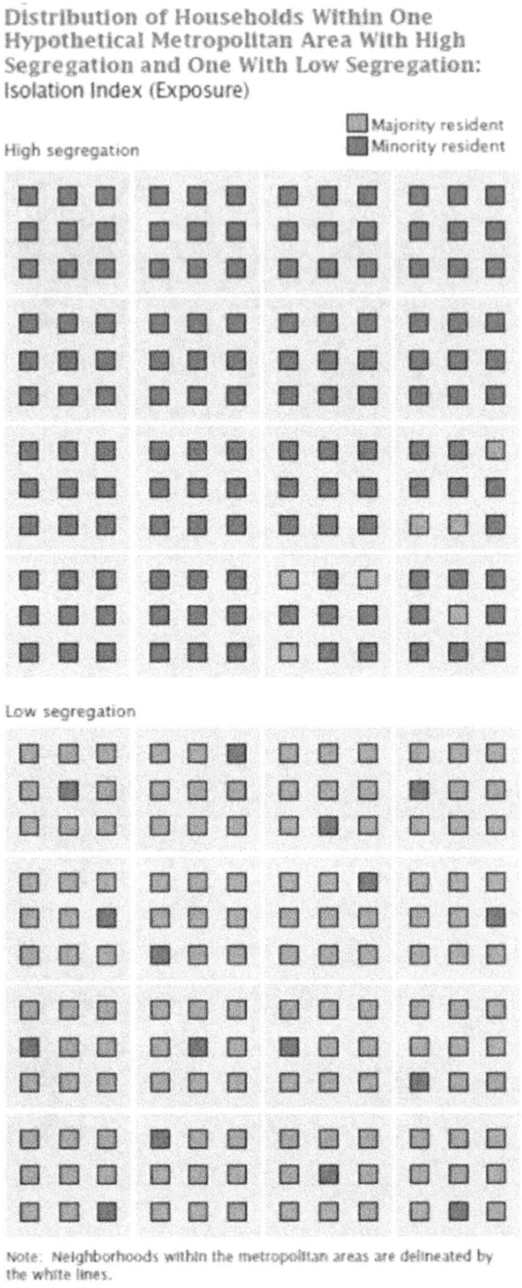

Fig. 9.4 Illustrations of segregation measures – isolation index (Iceland et al. 2002: 19)

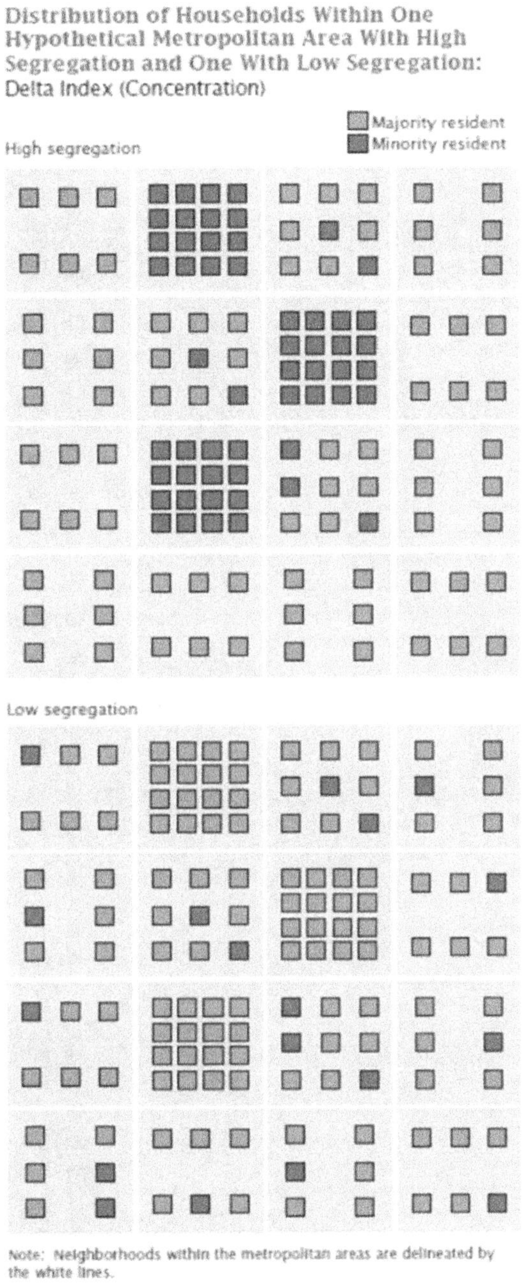

Fig. 9.5 Illustrations of segregation measures – delta index (Iceland et al. 2002:11)

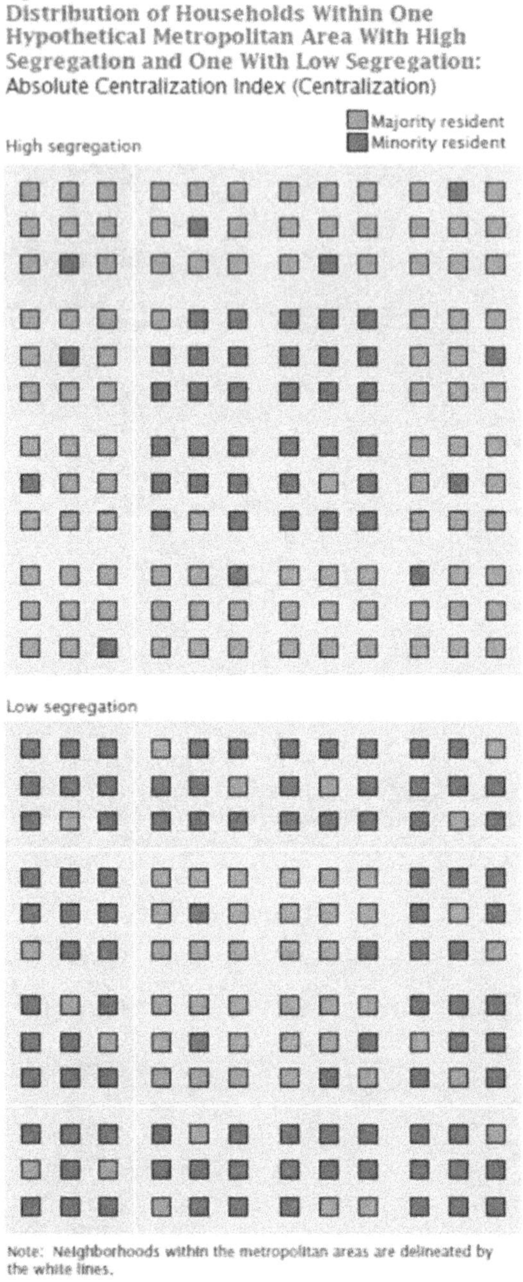

Fig. 9.6 Illustrations of segregation measures – absolute centralization index (Iceland et al. 2002: 12)

Fig. 9.7 Illustrations of segregation measures – spatial proximity index (Iceland et al. 2002: 13)

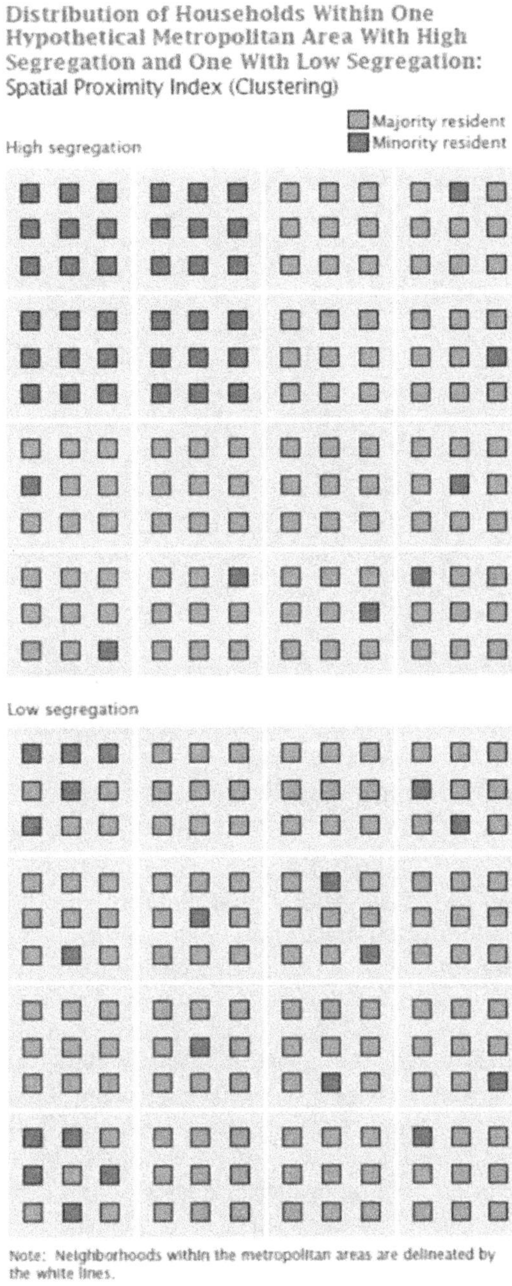

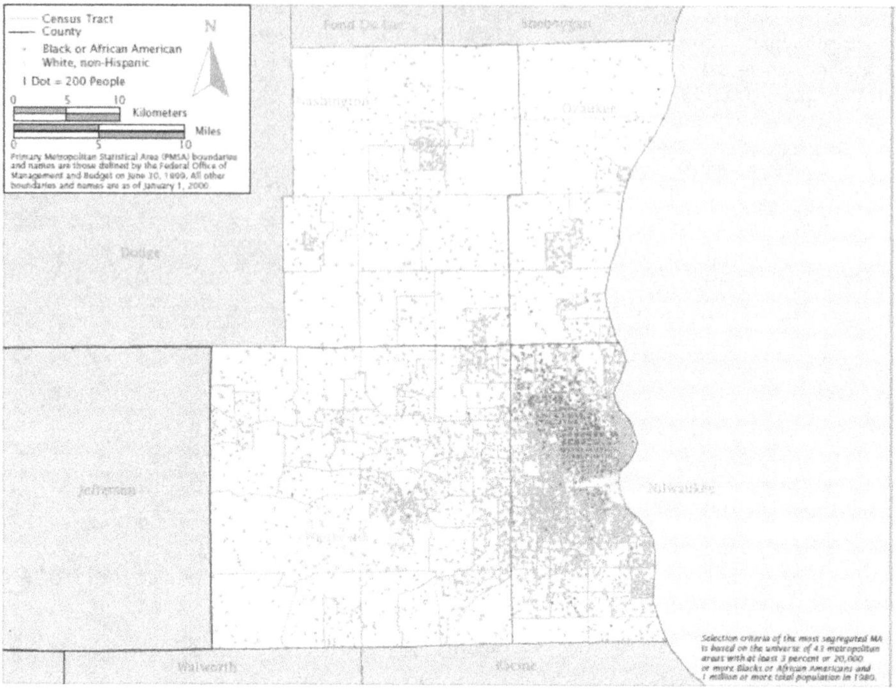

Fig. 9.8 Milwaukee-Waukesha, WI (Iceland et al. 2002: 70, originally from US Census Bureau)

9.3 Social Mobility

Social mobility takes one of two forms: intergenerational and intragenerational mobility. **Intergenerational mobility** refers to a change in social position (either upward or downward) of children in relation to their parents. **Intragenerational mobility** means a change in social position experienced during a person's life time. While the US is typically conceived of as 'the land of opportunity', it is relatively rare for a young person from a poor or working-class background to move into the upper middle class (Blau and Duncan 1967). As described above, the key factor for explaining this is educational attainment. A child's education is heavily influenced by their family's social status. In addition, parents, teachers, and peers impact the educational and career aspirations of the child, and these aspirations are critical to achieving educational and career goals throughout the child's life course. While we do observe some upward or downward social mobility, it is more common for people to move horizontally – they move from one job to another, at about the same social level. According to a recent study in the US, social mobility has been low; and given growing rates of inequality, the influence of parents has increased (Chetty et al. 2014).

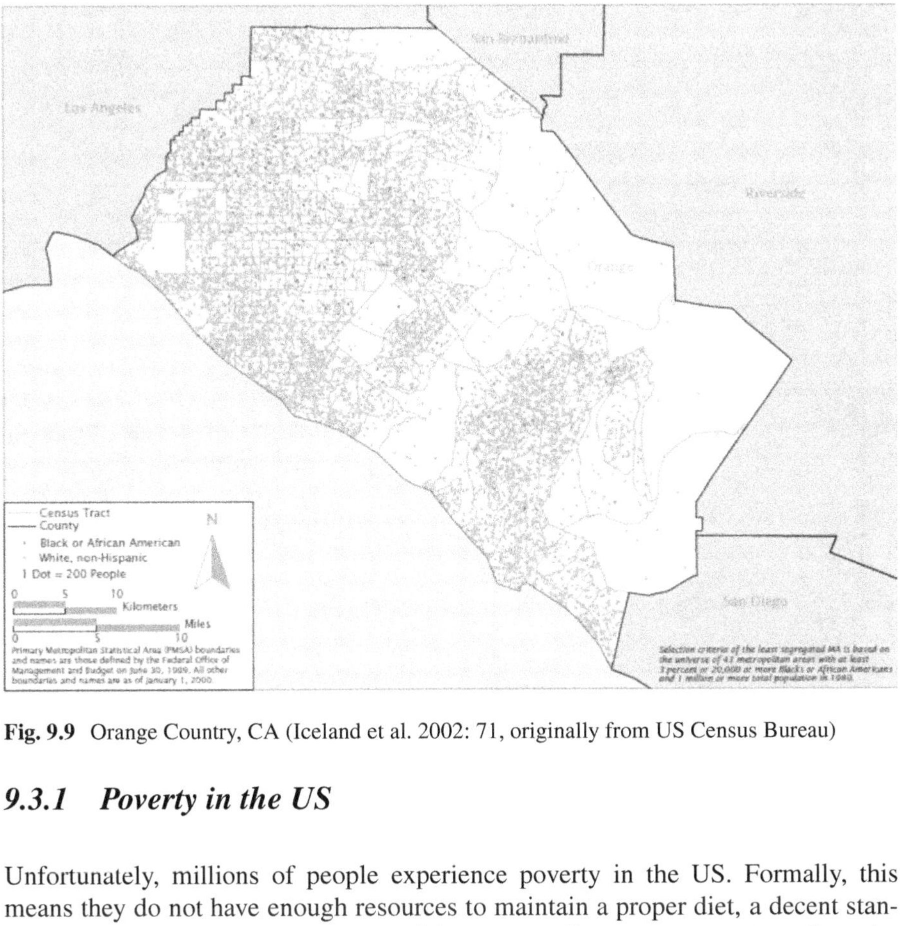

Fig. 9.9 Orange Country, CA (Iceland et al. 2002: 71, originally from US Census Bureau)

9.3.1 Poverty in the US

Unfortunately, millions of people experience poverty in the US. Formally, this means they do not have enough resources to maintain a proper diet, a decent standard of living, and healthy living conditions. According to a recent report from the US Census, the official poverty rate in 2015 was 13.5%, and 43.1 million people lived in poverty (Proctor et al. 2016).

The figure below (Fig. 9.10) shows how the absolute number and rate of poverty has changed over time.

As can be seen above, poverty declined substantially during the late 1960s and 1970s in both the total number of people and rate. Rates fluctuated over the 1980s and 1990s, and these numbers increased in late 2000 following an economic recession. Recently, rates have remained relatively high, and the 2015 poverty rate was slightly higher than in 2007, the year before the most recent "great recession".

Poverty is experienced differently across social groups by age, race/ethnicity, and gender. A report by Proctor et al. (2016) revealed that the poverty rate for children (age 18 and below) is 19.7%, which is much higher compared to the rate for those who are working ages (18–64), 12.4%. The poverty rate for the elderly

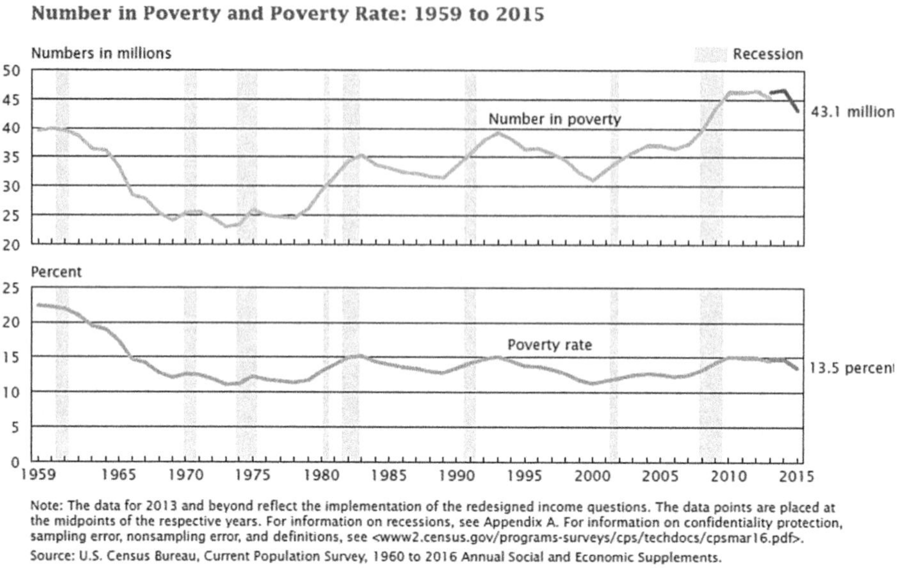

Fig. 9.10 Absolute numbers and rate of poverty over time (Proctor et al. 2016: 12)

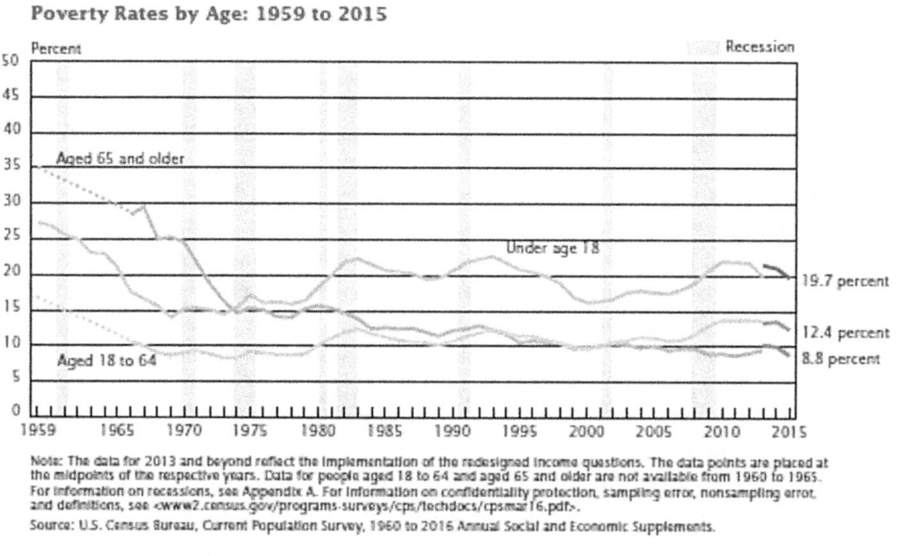

Fig. 9.11 Poverty rates by age: 1959–2015 (Proctor et al. 2016: 14)

(65 and above) has been consistently declining during the past decades, and it was 8.8% in 2015 (Fig. 9.11).

As for race and ethnicity, poverty is more common among non-Hispanic blacks (i.e. 24.1%) and Hispanics (i.e. 21.4%). Conversely, it is less common among non-

Hispanic whites (i.e. 9.1%) and Asians (i.e. 11.4%). In terms of gender, males are less likely to live in poverty than females (i.e. 12.2% for males vs. 14.8% for females), and this gap is largely driven by labor force activity among those in the working ages. Differences in poverty are most striking by educational attainment. As is shown, among those with a college degree, only 4.5% lived in poverty. However, 26.3% of people without a high school diploma lived in poverty.

9.3.2 Measures of Poverty

In order to measure poverty, the US Census follows the poverty threshold that the Office of Management and Budget's (OMB) Statistical Policy Directive 14 provides. This particular kind of measure is considered an *absolute measure* of poverty. The threshold is calculated based on cost estimates for families of different sizes and compositions. This is a very conservative estimate that has not been updated in many decades. For example, the cost estimate for family of four (i.e. two adults with two children under age 18) is $24,036 (or about $2000 a month) as of 2015, and thus a family of the four with an annual income lower than $24,036 is considered poor (Proctor et al. 2016).

This measure is often criticized as a measure of poverty status and differs from those used in other developed countries. Criticisms include the following:

- it does not take into account noncash forms of income available to the poor, such as food stamps, Medicaid, and public housing subsidies;
- it tends to overemphasize budget spent on food and underestimate the share spent on housing; and
- it underestimates health care costs, especially for the elderly who spend a relatively small proportion of their income on food, but often face more health issues.

9.3.3 Relative and Absolute Poverty

In defining poverty, it is useful to distinguish between relative poverty and absolute poverty. **Relative poverty** refers to a status of lacking resources *in relation to* those who have more, and it is more common in industrialized countries. By contrast, **absolute poverty** means a lack of enough food to eat and survive, which can be life threatening. Absolute poverty is more common in developing countries, and as was mentioned above, is also used in the US.

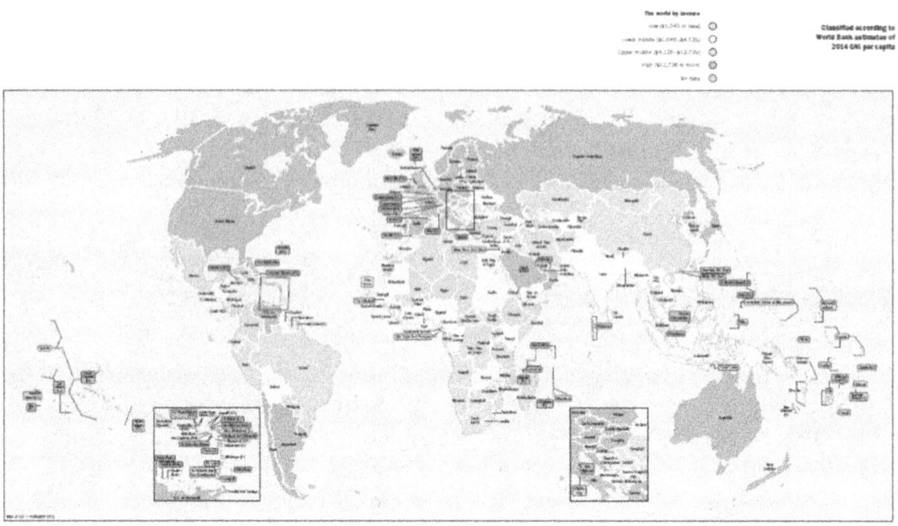

Fig. 9.12 World by income (World Bank 2016)

9.3.4 *Global Inequalities*

Global inequality refers to the systemic differences in wealth and power among countries (Giddens et al. 2016). The World Bank uses per person gross national income (GNI) to classify countries into four economic classes: high income, upper-middle income, lower-middle income and low income. The following map illustrates how this is globally distributed (Fig. 9.12).

As of 2017, high income countries have a GNI per capita greater than $12,475, and people in these countries enjoy the highest overall standards of living. There are 79 countries classified as high-income countries, and about 18% of the world's population resides in these high-income countries. However, their income makes up about 68% of the world total income (World Bank 2014). These countries include European countries, the US, Canada, and several Asian countries, such as Japan, Korea, Singapore, and Taiwan.

Middle-income countries (including both lower and upper middle) are mostly located in Asia (East, Southeast, and middle-East), North Africa, South America and Central America. In 108 (56 upper- and 52 lower-) middle-income countries, about 70% of world populations reside and command 31% of the total global income (World Bank 2014). Upper-middle-income and lower-middle-income countries are divided at a GNI per capita of $4035. The middle-income countries have begun to industrialize relatively late in twentieth century, and thus their living standards are not quite as high as the ones in the high-income countries. However, their living conditions are definitely better than the ones in the low-income countries.

Low-income countries have a GNI per capita lower than $1026 and 31 countries are classified in this category (World Bank 2017a). While they are primarily in east-

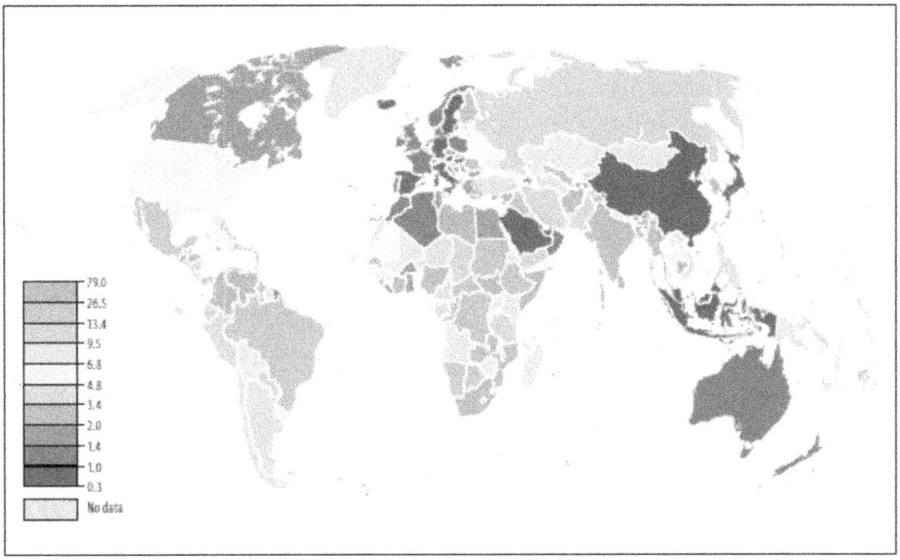

Fig. 9.13 Violent deaths per 100,000 residents per year, 2008–2012 (World Bank 2017b: 44)

ern, western, and sub-Saharan Africa, several countries are in Southeast Asia (e.g. Cambodia), East Asia (e.g. North Korea) and Caribbean (e.g. Haiti). Among the world population, about 12% of them reside in one of the low-income countries, but their income is only 0.7% of the world's total income (World Bank 2014). Additionally, this income inequality is growing as the population is growing faster in low-income countries with higher fertility rates, compared to population growth in other countries (Giddens et al. 2016).

Global income inequalities are also consistent with violence. The map below shows that violence is a major problem in low-income countries, such as Afghanistan, Somalia, and South Sudan, as well as some middle-income countries in America, including Mexico and Brazil (Fig. 9.13).

While more than 740,000 people die each year because of violence, the majority of these deaths are not due to ongoing wars. Rather, insufficient policy implementation, often combined with poor practices of the policies have been offered as primary reasons (World Bank 2017b) (Fig. 9.14).

Lower income countries also suffer from high levels of air pollution. As depicted in the above figure, the highest level of concentration of fine particulate matter is found among the middle-income countries. These countries have experienced rapid industrialization in recent years, yet sufficient policy to control pollution has not been adopted. The figure also shows that there have been steep increases in the levels of concentration of fine particulates in the past decade in both lower-middle income countries and low-income countries. Thus, it will be increasingly important to find ways to avoid the air pollution while pursuing economic development.

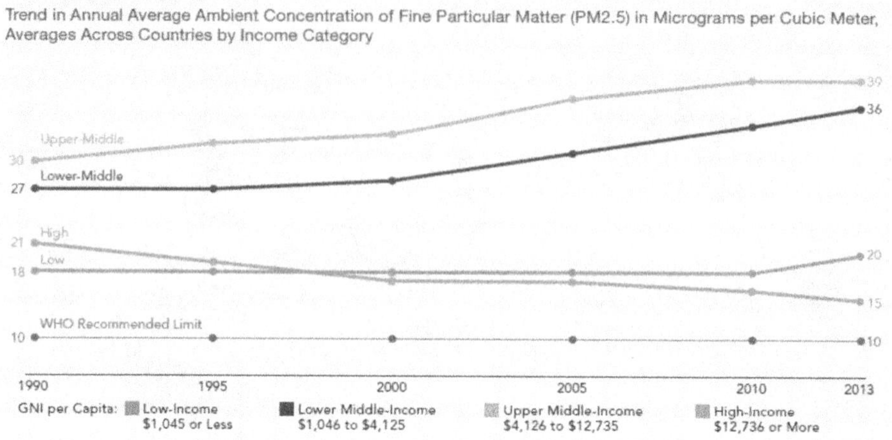

Fig. 9.14 Levels of air pollution (Population Reference Bureau 2016: 5)

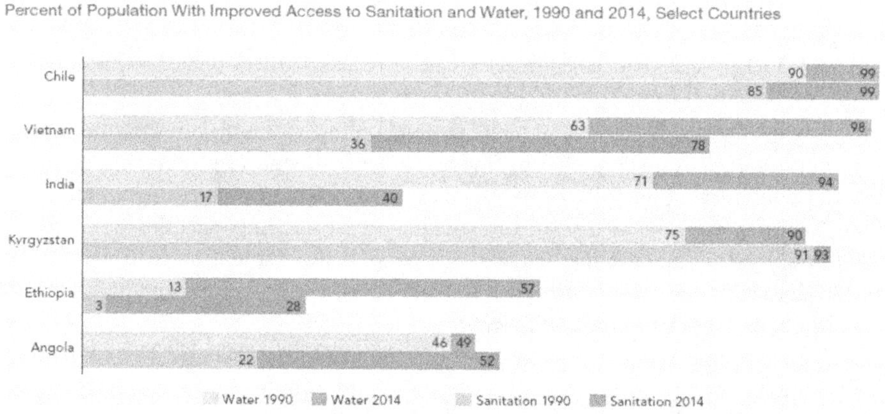

Fig. 9.15 Access to water and sanitation (Population Reference Bureau 2016: 7)

Global inequality also shapes health disparities across the world. People living in high-income countries are healthier, are less likely to suffer from disease, and live longer than those in low-income countries. For example, the average life expectancies among people in developed countries are 76 for men and 82 for women. However, they are 68 (for men) and 72 (for women) among those residing in less developed countries, and the life expectancies are even shorter for people in developing countries (i.e. 61 for men and 64 for women).

In recent years, more people in low-income countries have access to sanitation and water (see the below figure). However, despite the improvement, several countries still lack clean water and proper sanitation. Also, they are more likely to suffer from malnutrition and insufficient health care facilities (Fig. 9.15).

9.4 Social Structure and Individual Health

So far, we reviewed how social structures may place members of a society in different socioeconomic positions. While the link between social stratification and an individual's health outcomes may seem obvious, the debate of structure vs. agency in understanding an individual's health and disease has been a central question in medical sociology (Cockerham 2005).

Structures are "sets of mutually sustaining schemas and resources that empower or constrain social action and tend to be reproduced by that social action" (Sewell 1992: 19, recited from Cockerham 2005); and **agency** can be defined as "the temporally constructed engagement of actors of different structural environments" that reproduce and transform the structures (Emirbayer and Mische 1998: 970; Cockerham 2005). The relative emphasis on either structure or agency has led to the development of two frameworks: the *health belief model* and the *health lifestyle* model. According to **the health belief model**, some people adopt preventive health behaviors and some people don't, and the differences stem from varying degrees of health beliefs about: (1) susceptibility of particular health problem; (2) seriousness of the health problem; (3) possibility of lowering the risk of developing the health problem; and (4) feasibility of adopting preventive health behaviors (Becker 1974; Weitz 2007). The health belief model recognizes demographic characteristics (e.g. race/ethnicity, gender and age), psychosocial variables (e.g. personality characteristics), structural factors (e.g. access to the knowledge and resources), and the external environment (e.g. health campaigns), as factors affecting the beliefs. While incorporating social factors into individual's health decision making, the health belief model emphasizes *agency* as individuals makes choices for themselves – over *structure* that limits the choices available to individuals (Weitz 2007). The **health lifestyle theory**, on the other hand, emphasizes social group (i.e. structure) rather than individual (i.e. agency) behavior (Cockerham 2005). According to this model, an individual's healthy (or unhealthy) behavior is oriented by demographic characteristics (e.g. social class position, age, race/ethnicity, gender), cultural membership (e.g. religion), and living conditions (e.g. housing, neighborhood). These factors directly shape 'life chances' and indirectly affect 'life choices' through the socialization process. As shown in the figure below, life choices and life chances are intertwined as both come together to form habitual disposition to act, which may lead to action and in turn health lifestyles (reproduction) (Fig. 9.16).

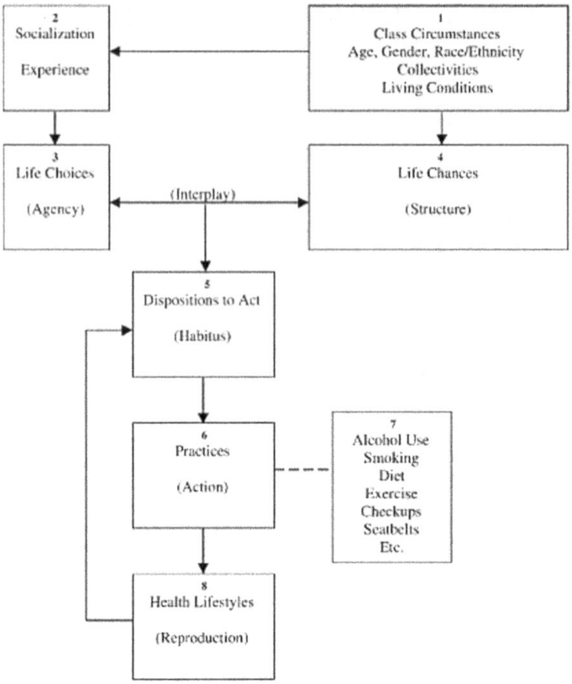

Fig. 9.16 Health lifestyle theory (Cockerham 2005: 57)

Resources, Links, and Recommended Readings

Readings on the Inverse Care Law and Fundamental Causes of Disease

Hart, J. 1971. "The Inverse Care Law." *The Lancet*, February 27: 405–412.

Link, B. G., & Phelan, J. 1995. "Social Conditions as Fundamental Causes of Diseases." *Journal of Health and Social Behavior*, 36: 80–94.

Activities and Discussion Questions

Activity 1: Create a conceptual model to describe mechanisms through which social class influences individual's health. In your model, include education, occupation and income for social class measures, as well as other mediators you can think of, such as marriage, employment, health behaviors, and access to health care, and use arrows to indicate the direction of influence from one variable to another.

Activity 2: Is universal health care necessary? Divide the class into two groups based on students' answer to the question, and debate whether the government or individuals should be responsible for health care.

Discussion Question 1: Describe the trend of social mobility in the US, and discuss whether and how it may differ by race and ethnicity. Think about whether racial and ethnic differentials in social mobility will be growing, declining or stay stable, and explain why.

Discussion Question 2: Recently, *The Economist* published the glass-ceiling index for 29 OECD countries (http://www.economist.com/blogs/graphicdetail/2017/03/daily-chart-0), based on 10 indicators including higher education, workforce participation, pay, child-care costs, maternity and paternity rights, business-school applications, and representation in senior jobs. The index estimates chances of equal treatment in the workplace, and the United States ranked 20 with below 60%, implying the chance of equal treatment in the workplace is lower than 60%. Discuss how the social status of women may influence gender inequality in health.

Discussion Question 3: Describe patterns and explanations of poverty in the US, and explain why poverty among children has increased.

Key Terms

- **Social Class**: socioeconomic variations in their material prosperity and power, often measured by income, wealth, education and occupation
- **Social Stratification**: systematic inequalities between groups of people
- **Ascribed Status**: the status people are born with
- **Achieved Status**: the status people earn
- **Meritocracy**: a social stratification system based on personal merit, such as a person's knowledge, skills and effort
- **Class Consciousness**: a belief that working class people will recognize their needs in opposition to those valued in capitalist societies, which will lead to revolution
- **False Consciousness**: the state in which classes are unaware of their subordinate position and thus prevented from organizing on the basis of their true interest
- **Social Status**: the position that a person occupies in the social order
- **Social Power**: one's ability to enact change, control resources, command decisions
- **Occupational Prestige**: prestige that some occupations offer
- **Segregation**: the physical and social separation of people by certain categories, often measured by
  - **Evenness**: the differential distribution of the population of interest
  - **Exposure**: the degree of potential contact or possibility of interaction between minority and majority group members
  - **Concentration**: the relative amount of physical space occupied by a minority group in the metropolitan area
  - **Centralization**: the degree to which a group is spatially located near the center of an urban area
  - **Clustering**: the extent to which areal units inhabited by minority members adjoin to another or cluster in space
- **Social Mobility**: takes one of two forms
  - Intergenerational mobility: a change in social position (either upward or downward) of children in relation to their parents

  - Intragenerational mobility: a change in social position experienced during a person's life time

- **Poverty**: a status when people do not have enough resources to maintain a proper diet, a decent standard of living, and healthy living conditions
- **Relative Poverty**: a status of lacking resources in relation to those who have more
- **Absolute Poverty**: a status of lacking enough food to eat and survive
- **Global Inequality**: the systemic differences in wealth and power among countries
- **Structures**: sets of mutually sustaining schemas and resources that empower or constrain social action and tend to be reproduced by that social action
- **Agency**: the temporally constructed engagement of actors of different structural environments that reproduce and transform the structures
- **Health Belief Model**: a framework developed to understand roles of individuals in health behaviors focusing, emphasizing agency over structure
- **Health Lifestyle Model**: a framework developed to understand roles of structures in health behaviors, emphasizing structure over agency

Study Questions

Describe the role of social status and power as it relates to life chances.

***Example Exam Question:** "Based upon the passage, what would be the most plausible hypothesis for a study evaluating the effect of socioeconomic status (SES) on the likelihood of alcohol dependence?

A. Factors that reflect disadvantaged SES will increase the probability of alcohol dependence among those with the high-risk genotype on GABRA2.
B. Factors related to SES will affect the probability of alcohol dependence only when matched with gender and GABRA2 genotype.
C. Factors related to SES will have no effect on the probability of alcohol dependence among those with either high- or low-risk genotype on GABRA2.
D. Factors that reflect advantaged SES will decrease the probability of alcohol dependence among those with the high-risk genotype on *GABRA2*." (AAMC 2012: 120)

*For more information, visit https://students-residents.aamc.org/applying-medical-school/article/whats-mcat-exam/

References

AAMC. (2012). *Preview guide for the MCAT2015 exam* (2nd ed.). American Association of Medical Colleges: Washington D.C.

Becker, M. H. (1974). *The health belief model and personal health behavior*. San Francisco: Society for Public Health Education.

Blau, P. M., & Duncan, O. D. (1967). *The American occupational structure*. New York: Wiley.

Chetty, R., Hendren, N., Kline, P., Saez, E., & Turner, N. (2014). Is the United States still a land of opportunity? recent trends in intergenerational mobility. *American Economic Review Papers and Proceedings, 104*(5), 141–147.

Cockerham, W. (2005). Health lifestyle theory and the convergence of agency and structure. *Journal of Health and Social Behavior, 46*, 51–67.

Coser, L. (1977). *Masters of sociological thought: Ideas in historical and social context* (2nd ed.). Long Grove: Waveland Press.

Emirbayer, M., & Mische, A. (1998). What is sgency? *American Journal of Sociology, 103*, 962–1023.

Giddens, A., Duneier, M., Appelbaum, R. P., & Carr, D. (2016). *Introduction to sociology* (10th ed.). New York City: W.W. Norton & Company.

Iceland, J., Weinberg, D. H., & Steinmetz, E., (2002). Racial and ethnic residential segregation in the United States: 1980–2000.U.S. Census Bureau, Series CENSR-3, U.S. Census Bureau, Government Printing Office, Washington, DC. Retrieved from the website at: https://www.census.gov/hhes/www/housing/housing_patterns/pdf/censr-3.pdf

Massey, D. S., & Denton, N. A. (1988). The dimensions of residential segregation. *Social Forces, 67*, 281–315.

Macionis, J. J. (2014). *Sociology* (15th ed.) ed.). Upper Saddle River: Pearson.

Population Reference Bureau. (2016). *2016 World Population Data Sheet*. Retrieved from the website at: http://www.prb.org/Publications/Datasheets/2016/2016-world-population-data-sheet.aspx.

Proctor, B. D., & Kollar, M. A. (2016). *Income and Poverty in the United States: 2015: Current Population Reports*, P60-256(RV), U.S. Census Bureau, Government Printing Office, Washington, DC. Retrieved from the website at: https://www.census.gov/content/dam/Census/library/publications/2016/demo/p60-256.pdf

Ritzer, G., & Michael Ryan, J. (2010). *The concise encyclopedia of sociology*. Chichester: Wiley-Blackwell.

Sewell, W. H. (1992). A theory of structure: Duality, agency, and transformation. *American Journal of Sociology, 98*, 1–29.

US Bureau of Labor Statistics. 2015. Women in the Labor Force: A databook.. Retrieved from the website at https://www.bls.gov/opub/reports/womens-databook/archive/women-in-the-labor-force-a-databook-2015.pdf.

US Department of Education. (2013). *Digest of Education Statistics*. Retrieved from the website at: https://nces.ed.gov/programs/digest/d13/tables/dt13_211.60.asp.

US Department of Education. (2015). *Digest of Education Statistics*. Retrieved from the website at: https://nces.ed.gov/programs/digest/d15/tables/dt15_219.46.asp.

Weber, M. (1922). *Economy and society*. Berkeley: University of California Press.

Weitz, R. (2007). *The sociology of health, illness, and health care*. Belmont: Thompson Higher Education.

World Bank. (2014). *World development report 2014: Risk and opportunity: Managing risk for development*. Retrieved from the website at http://siteresources.worldbank.org/EXTNWDR2013/Resources/8258024-1352909193861/8936935-1356011448215/8986901-1380046989056

World Bank. (2016). World Development Indicators. Retrieved from the website at: http://data.worldbank.org/products/wdi-maps.

World Bank. (2017a). *World Bank Country and Lending Groups*. Retrieved from the website at: https://datahelpdesk.worldbank.org/knowledgebase/articles/906519.

World Bank. (2017b). *World Development Report*. Retrieved from the website at: http://www.worldbank.org/en/publication/wdr2017

Chapter 10
Health, Health Care and Health Disparities

Objectives

- Understand medicine as a social institution.
- Understand the causes and consequences of health disparities by race, class, and gender.
- Understand the causes and consequences of health care disparities by race, class and gender.

Foundational Concept 9
"*Cultural and social differences influence well-being...*

Social structure and demographic factors influence peoples' health and well-being. Knowledge about basic sociological theories, social institutions, culture and demographic characteristics of societies is important to understand, [as is the ability to understand] how they shape peoples' lives and their daily interactions...

Content Category 9A focuses on the link between social structures and human interactions." (AAMC 2015: 255)

Foundational Concept 10

"*Social stratification and access to resources influence well-being...*

Social stratification and inequality affect all human societies, and shape the lives of all individuals by affording privileges to some and positioning others at a disadvantage...

Content Category 10A focuses on a broad understanding of social class, including theories of social stratification, social mobility, and poverty." (AAMC 2015: 259)

G. Garcia-Alexander et al., *Social Foundations of Behavior for the Health Sciences*,
DOI 10.1007/978-3-319-64950-4_10

10.1 Health and Medicine

The institution of **medicine** consists of all the health care providers, hospitals and other facilities that deliver medical care. Doctors and other health care professionals address the health needs of individual patients by understanding their symptoms, coming to a diagnosis, and providing treatment. Many sociologists also work in the context of medicine. Unlike health care providers who are interested in the needs of individual patients, sociologists are interested in the social causes and consequences of health and illness. This means understanding how individuals experience health and illness, and how those experiences reflect cultural and social structure rather than just specific disease processes. Sociologists are also interested in patterns of diseases and how they are spread across different groups in society. Both health care professionals and medical sociologists usually define health in the same way. The most commonly accepted definition of health comes from the World Health Organization: **health** is "a state of complete physical, mental and social well-being and not merely the absence of disease or infirmity" (Grad 2002: 981).

10.1.1 Illness Experience

To a sociologist, a diagnosis is not simply a private individual experience. It is often the beginning of a social process in which a subjective label is applied to someone. That label both affects how others see them, and how they see themselves. As described in Chap. 3, there are social and cultural expectations about someone who has been diagnosed with an illness. The sick role includes that set of expectations and responsibilities associated with being sick. The person is not held responsible for failing to carry out their normal duties, however, they are also required to take specific action to get better. They must seek competent medical help, and comply with treatment. Failure to carry out the sick role faithfully could cause others to label that person as someone who is feigning illness to get out of their responsibilities. There are, however, a number of critiques of the sick role. What happens when a person contracts HIV or lung cancer? Regardless of whether they comply with treatment, they still may be held responsible for their illness and stigmatized. The sick role also fails to take into account the social and economic circumstances of the patient. Non-unionized workers are much less likely to take work off than unionized workers (Kurani et al. 2017). Therefore, even with a legitimate illness, they are unable to take time off work for financial reasons.

Whether or not a person is considered ill or well is not always a simple matter of biology or getting a medical diagnosis. Whether someone is considered sick in many cases depends on the culture, the time and place in which they live. **Medicalization** refers to the increasing tendency to treat problems previously defined as non-medical, in medical terms. Drug abuse is a classic example of medicalization. A few decades ago, drug abuse was seen as a personal failing, or a deviant behavior. It wasn't a matter for doctors. However, now it is defined as a medical condition, carries a medical diagnosis and can often be treated in a medical setting with pharmaceutical treatment. Drug abuse may provide a positive example of medicalization because many people are able to overcome addiction and live their lives as a result of medical treatment.

There are also a number of negative examples of medicalization. One such example is when illness is inappropriately medicalized by drug companies seeking to increase profits by marketing a "cure" to the public and their health care providers. Attention deficit hyperactivity disorder more commonly known as ADHD is such an example. According to the National Center for Health Statistics (2014) the number of children under 18 on stimulants to treat ADHD and other behavior problems has increased from less than 1% to more than 4% since 1988. This fivefold increase in medication is not likely to be caused by a dramatic increase in rates of ADHD, sociologists would point out it more likely corresponds to the creation of a new market for drug companies. On one-hand, there are cases where children are unable to function, and benefit from medication. On the other hand, since there is no biological marker for ADHD, the disease is diagnosed based on teachers' and parents' perceptions of child behavior. The dramatic increase in medicating children corresponds with social factors like the need for children to sit for long hours in school.

In the case of both drug abuse and ADHD, the benefits of medicalization include reducing stigma and providing access to effective treatments. Individuals with medical conditions aren't labeled as bad, but instead they are seen as sick, requiring medicine, and eligible to adopt the sick role and thus be relieved of accountability for their illness. On the other hand, medicalization also diverts attention from structural explanations. The problems associated with ADHD may be more a result of school systems that expect young children to be still for long periods of time, even if that is neither possible, nor desirable for many children.

10.2 Health Disparities

Social epidemiology is the study of the social and environmental causes and consequences of disease. Social epidemiologists seek to understand how race, class, and gender as well as the social and physical environment influence people's health throughout their life.

Health is not distributed equally across the population. Social class, which includes education, income and occupation play an important role in health status. Specifically, those with more education have higher incomes, more prestigious occupations, and live longer and healthier lives. This is something we all know intuitively, but don't often consider why it's the case. In order to illustrate this point, Michael Marmot (2004) asks his readers to imagine a parade in which we line up people according to their level of education. We begin with those who dropped out of school because they were unable, or unwilling to complete it. Then the high school graduates, those who went to community college, and those with college degrees. Finally, those with graduate degrees, the Masters, the Ph.D.s, and the M.D.s. "As the parade progresses, we note the changes in style and demeanor, of comportment and confidence, and of increasing affluence. We notice something else: a healthy glow, increasing in radiance with those going past. If we could but measure this glow, it would show us that this sorting of people according to their education has also, in a remarkably precise manner, sorted them according to their health and length of life" (2004, pp. 14–15). Any of us can imagine this parade. And if we repeat this parade, but instead of education we sort people by income, we will get exactly the same result. This is not surprising of course, since there is much overlap between people with a lot of education and those with high incomes. Doctors make more money than teachers, and teachers make more money than grocery store clerks. Each increase in level of education, brings with it increases in income, and usually, a better job with more flexible hours, better benefits, and even better working conditions, all of which contribute to health.

When considering the impact of social class on health, the common explanation is that the poor are poor because of some individual failings like laziness or lack of willpower, and it is those failings that explain their frequent unemployment, their poor nutrition, or their tendency to smoke. This is a tempting explanation because people with less education are out of work more often, do have worse nutrition, and are more likely to smoke. However, pointing the finger at individual explanations for health differences only explains the more proximate cause. It does not explain *why* joblessness, poor nutrition, and smoking are more likely to occur among the poor. In other words, individual behavior doesn't really explain the link between class and health. For example, rich smokers live longer than poor smokers, so it's *not* just the smoking. So how do we answer the question, *why does having less education and income lead to poor health?*

10.2.1 Social Class and Health

The effects of social class on health begin in early life, with early childhood experience (Zimmerman et al. 2015). Poor mothers who lack proper nutrition and medical care, and live in stressful living conditions, are more likely to have pre-term children and children with low birth weight. Both of these factors have been shown to have lifelong consequences for learning, and even illness in adulthood. Poor children are also more likely to grow up in homes with high levels financial strain because their parents have more difficulty staying employed, keeping stable housing, and having enough food. All of these things contribute to stress in the home that affects children's cognitive development, immune systems, and ability to do well in school. Outside of the home, both neighborhood and school characteristics also contribute to a lifelong risk of poor health. As discussed in Chap. 5, schools in poor neighborhoods also have fewer resources, which means that kids in low-income families also have less access to a high quality education. Poor neighborhoods also often lack safe places to play outside which can decrease exercise and increase risk of obesity.

Low income neighborhoods are also characterized by increased risk of violent crime and homicide.

10.2.2 Education and Health

As a fundamental cause of poor health, education is a resource that can be used to avoid health risks and lessen the impacts of disease (Link and Phelan 1995). Education provides direct benefits, like the ability to think critically, understand information about health risks and nutrition, and in short, make better choices in life. However, much of the impact of education on health is indirect. People with more education are likely to earn more income and have better jobs throughout their life. Having more income means having access to many of the resources that social epidemiologists have found to influence both health and life expectancy. People with more education are less likely to become unemployed, more likely to have access to adequate nutrition, and are more likely to live in high quality neighborhoods. They are also more likely to have the kinds of jobs that provide health insurance which allows them to take better care of themselves throughout their life. Education also influences health behaviors. People with more education are more likely to exercise, have better nutrition, and less likely to smoke. Improved health behaviors, like nutrition may be a direct result of education. However, having more financial resources is also necessary to have access to higher quality food. As for smoking, research shows that virtually everyone knows that smoking causes lung disease and cancer. However, people with less education have more stressful lives, which can make it more difficult to quit smoking, and also have less access to health care resources to help quit. Finally, having more education means having social networks that can provide resources in times of need. People with more education also have the kinds of social ties including friends, neighbors, and coworkers that can make a difference for your health.

The links between education and health are so strong, that a common phrase among social scientists is: "education policy is health policy." When considering funding for education, politicians do not often make a strong association between education and health. However, since health care costs are much higher among people with less education, failing to fund educational programs that benefit low income families not only has a negative impact on the quality of schools, but it also has a negative impact on our health care system as well.

10.2.3 Occupation and Health

Occupation is also a significant social determinant of health. People with higher paying and more prestigious jobs enjoy better health and longer lives than people with lower paying, hourly jobs requiring little education. There are two different ways that occupation affects health. The first way that occupation affects health is that many jobs, especially those that require little education, tend to be more physically hazardous jobs in the trades, manufacturing, construction, and truck driving as well as jobs in the service industry. These jobs carry relatively high risk of injury, exposure to chemicals, and exposure to difficult working conditions like heat and noise. All of these work characteristics carry negative health consequences and partly explain why people with better jobs have better health. These jobs can also be psychologically damaging. People with more dangerous jobs not only have higher rates of illness related to exposure to chemicals, but they also have higher rates of cardio-vascular disease that may be related to the stress of having to constantly be on the lookout for danger (Kivimäki and Kawachi 2015).

The second way that jobs affect health is through increased psychological stress associated with a mismatch between the demands of a job, and the amount of control one has over the work. The lower a person is on the career ladder, the more likely it is that they have both a demanding boss, and little opportunity for creative input, or control over their work environment including their working hours, where the work occurs, or even how the work gets done. This is why people with lower occupational prestige tend to be less healthy. It's not just the money, it's also the fact that you are not able to exert any personal control and that causes psychological stress. When experienced day in and day out occupational stress leads to weakened immune functioning, high blood pressure and heart disease. The bottom line is that a sense of control matters. A similar health effect occurs with jobs that have little connection between effort and reward. If the job you occupy has little in the way of rewards, either financial or psychological, this causes the same kind of stress as lack of control, with the same health damaging effects.

10.2.4 Gender and Health

As Fig. 10.1 shows women of all races live longer than men of the same race. This has not always been true. Prior to the twentieth century, mostly because of childbirth, women's life expectancy was shorter than men's. However, owing to improved social status and increased health care access, women now have a lifespan that is about 5 years longer than men. Scientists are not exactly sure why that is the case, but there are two generally accepted explanations, one rooted in sex (biology) and other rooted in gender (social norms). The biological explanation is that female sex hormones have a protective effect on women's health. The sociological explanation is that gender norms preclude women from engaging in dangerous behavior like violence, or driving under the influence. It is likely that both are true and together explain women's longer life spans.

Although women live longer, they are more likely to suffer from illness throughout their lives. Again, scientists are not sure why, but here too, there are explanations rooted in both sex, and gender. The explanation based on sex is that they are more likely to experience illness because of hormones. However, women are also more

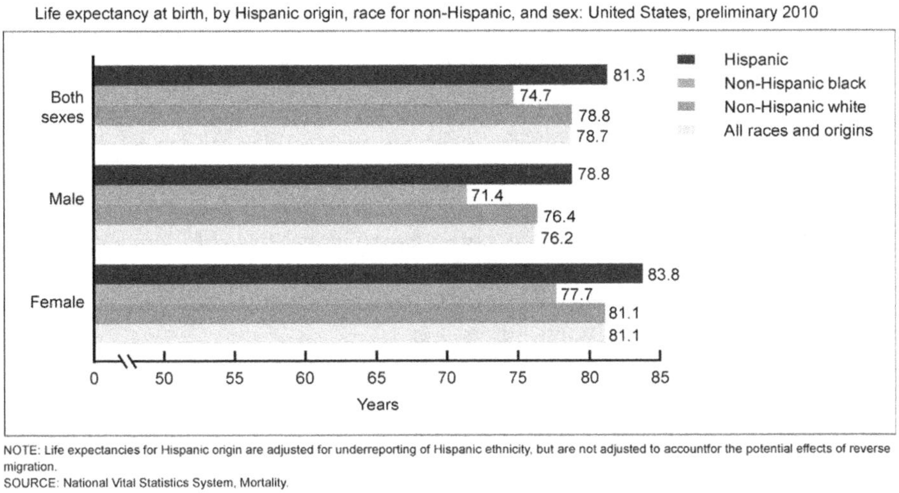

Fig. 10.1 Life expectancy at birth by race, ethnicity, and sex

likely to be employed in occupations characterized by high demands and low control; high effort, and low reward. Women are also disproportionately responsible for the second-shift, the care for children and home after the workday. The increased demands and little personal control afforded by women in society may explain increased risk of illness. A recent analysis, however, showed that between 1974 and 2004, women in the United States experienced improved health status. And these improvement could be explained in large part because of gains in education, employment and income (Schnittker 2007).

10.2.5 Racial and Ethnic Health Disparities

In the 6-month period following the terrorist attacks of 9/11, pregnant Muslim women in California experienced an increase in pre-term births and low-birthweight babies compared to the 6 months before 9/11. This increase was not found in other ethnic groups (Lauderdale 2006). The most likely cause of worsened pregnancy outcomes among Muslims was the negative psychological effects of experiencing the pervasive anti-Muslim sentiment of the time. More recent studies of young Black and Hispanic children who experience racial discrimination on social media also demonstrate increased depression and anxiety. These studies provide striking examples of how racism, prejudice, and discrimination get under the skin and cause physical and psychological illness in racial and ethnic minorities (Williams et al. 2010).

African Americans experience considerable health disparities. Infant mortality rates are more than twice as high than Whites, and life expectancy for a black male is 10 years shorter than for a White female (see Fig. 10.1). African Americans also have significantly higher rates of most of the leading causes of death including heart disease, strokes, cancer, diabetes, HIV, and homicide. There are several contributing factors to health disparities among African Americans and all of them can be traced to the historical and current experiences of racism and discrimination. Many African Americans report experiencing discrimination in their daily lives. Studies show that Black job applicants with similar qualifications are less likely to get the same jobs as White applicants (Williams 2010). There is continuing evidence of police profiling African Americans as well. The physical and psychological effects of experiencing racism on a daily basis in society contribute to higher rates of illness, especially cardiovascular disease and early death. The result of increased stress hormones in the body that over time accumulate and negatively affect health through elevated risk of high blood pressure and heart disease.

Another set of pathways involves the same set of factors related to social class described above. These emanate from persistent historical residential and educational segregation and discrimination in employment and the criminal justice system. As described in Chap. 5, both residential and educational segregation continue to result in increased risk of living in concentrated poverty and unequal access to education. The continuing legacy of societal racism results in persistent unequal treatment that leads to each of the risk factors associated with social class including early life factors, education, and occupational effects.

Health disparities among Hispanics are much more complicated. Hispanics, on average, have rates of infant mortality that are roughly equal to Whites and much lower than Native American or African Americans. Hispanics also have longer life expectancies that of all other racial and ethnic groups except for Asians (see Fig. 10.1). Since Hispanics have rates of poverty similar to African Americans, have low graduation rates, and are more likely than Whites to lack health insurance, the fact that they have better health status is difficult to understand. In fact, it has been called the "Hispanic Paradox." There are two different explanations for their better health profile. The "salmon bias" explanation suggests that Latino immigrants who become ill, or very old return to their country of origin to die. This means that many of the deaths of Latinos are not recorded in official statistics in the U.S. making their death rates look artificially lower. The second explanation is the "healthy immigrant" explanation. This explanation suggests that because immigrating is difficult and does not happen randomly, only the healthiest people come to the U.S, which also artificially inflates the health profile of Hispanic immigrants relative to U.S. born Hispanics and Whites. However, partly because of acculturation (see Chap. 5 for more information), Hispanic paradox is less salient (or becomes dismissive) among the higher generations: First generation immigrants are healthier than their children (2nd generation) and their grandchildren (3rd generation). As Hispanic immigrants are acculturated, they tend to lose positive cultural support systems, and more likely to engage in unhealthy risk behaviors, like drug and alcohol use and smoking, associated with poverty, stress, and U.S. culture. Another important factor to consider with the worsening health of Hispanics in the U.S. over time is the effect of being a minority. Hispanic immigrants often report prejudice and discrimination which has negative health effects.

Asian Americans have even better health indicators than both Hispanics, and Whites. At 86.5 years, life expectancy for Asian Americans is the longest of all racial/ethnic groups. However, there are large differences in the health profiles of various Asian American subgroups. In general, Chinese, Japanese, and Filipino immigrants all have lower death rates, longer life expectancy, and lower infant mortality than more recent immigrants from Southeast Asian countries, like Vietnam, or the Pacific Islands (Hawaii, Sumoa, Guam). And, like Hispanics, immigrants not born in the U.S. have better health indicators than their U.S. born children and grandchildren.

Native American health is much harder to track because they are often misclassified as White. However, what is known about Native American health indicators is they experience significant health disparities. The life expectancy of Native Americans is 76.9 years, placing them between African Americans and Whites. Rates of infant mortality follow the same general pattern, with rates better than African Americans, but worse than other race/ethnic groups. There are distinct differences in health profiles, however. Native Americans have the highest rates of death for accidental injuries, are twice as likely to die from diabetes, and three times more likely to die from liver disease. Chronic drug and alcohol abuse is epidemic in native populations. These excess death rates can be explained, in large part, by historic discrimination. Specifically, both geographic segregation on reservations, and lack of access to education, employment, and health care.

10.3 The Health Setting

10.3.1 Delivery of Health Care

The United States Health Care System is characterized by unequal access. Some people have access to all of the medical care they need, while many others have little or no access. In 2013, the year before the Affordable Care Act (sometimes referred to as "Obamacare") was implemented, more than 48 million people, (16% of the U.S. population) had no health insurance. In addition, many people who had insurance weren't able to use it because the out-of-pocket costs were too high, a problem known as underinsurance. It's perhaps surprising then that overuse of health care is also a significant problem in the U.S. Patients with health insurance, including those over 65 years old with Medicare, have more days in the hospital, office visits and medication than are medically necessary (Bodenheimer and Grumbach 2016). That is, compared to people with similar conditions, patients who use more care are not better off than those who use less. Don Berwick estimated that the cost of overuse was more than $550 billion dollars per year (Berwick and Hackbarth 2012).

Table 10.1 Health care payment types

Source of payment	Percent of population 2015 (%)
Uninsured	9
Private Insurance	
Individual Private Insurance	16
Employment-Based Insurance	56
Public Insurance	
Medicaid	20
Medicare	16
Military and Veterans	5

Note: Percents do not total to 100% because people can have more than one type of coverage
Source: U.S. Census Burea. Health Insurance Coverage in the United States: 2015 September 13, 2016 Report Number: P60-257 Jessica C. Barnett and Marina Vornovitsky

10.3.2 How Do We Pay for Care?

There are four ways that health care is paid for in the U.S.: out-of-pocket, individual insurance, employer-based insurance, and government programs including Medicare (covers the elderly and disabled), Medicaid (covers people with low incomes), and military insurance (Table 10.1).

Some uninsured people pay for health care out-of-pocket, but because health care is so expensive, very few people can afford to pay this way, and those that do report high levels of financial distress. In 2013, self-pay represented only about 13% of health expenditures in the US (Bodenheimer and Grumbach 2016). Individual private insurance is also a very small amount of the total, although it now covers twice as many adults and children as it did just 2 years ago before the Affordable Care Act was implemented. Among the provisions of the Affordable Care Act, is the *individual mandate*, which requires all citizens to purchase health insurance. For people with low incomes who can't afford to pay the premiums, there are government subsidies that help cover the cost. Critics argue that the mandate is an unnecessary government intrusion into private affairs, and people should not be forced to pay for insurance, especially if they don't need or want it. The reason it was enacted, however, was to make sure that all people who use health care pay their fair share. If only a few people who need to use health care services pay premiums, and large numbers of people don't pay, then the premiums will be much more costly than if everybody pays something. It also helps to prevent cost-shifting from the uninsured to the insured. Because uninsured people often end up in the hospital or emergency room, and do not pay for their care, the costs of those services are shifted onto paying patients, usually people with private or employer sponsored insurance. The mandate is a way to prevent the shifting of health care costs from the uninsured to those who do pay insurance.

Employer-based coverage is the dominant form of insurance coverage in the United States, and is a byproduct of our unique history and culture. During World War II, companies were not able to increase workers' wages because of government instituted wage controls. In order to provide incentives for recruitment and retention of employees, employers began offering insurance benefits. Over time this became an expectation of employees and now covers more than half of the U.S. population. It's important to recognize that employer based-insurance does not just represent a private transaction between an employer and an insurance company. The government subsidizes more than 250 billion dollars each year by allowing companies and individuals to write off the cost of insurance on their taxes (Gruber 2010). Even private, employer-sponsored insurance has a long history of being supported by government funding.

The final mechanism for paying health care costs is government-sponsored insurance. In 1965, the Medicare Act established both Medicare, the program that pays for elderly and disabled, and Medicaid, the program that pays for low-income individuals. A second provision of the ACA was to expand the Medicaid programs. Prior to 2014, most Medicaid programs required families to earn very low wages, well below poverty level. Under the ACA, all Americans earning up to 138% of federal poverty level would be eligible for Medicaid. This was another way to ensure that low income families who have historically been uninsured, would have access to medical care. Medicare covers mostly people over the age of 65, but it also covers some people with disabilities. Contrary to popular belief, undocumented individuals have never been eligible for government sponsored healthcare and rates of fraud are extremely low. Most undocumented workers and other immigrants do not attempt to sign up for public benefits for fear of being caught and deported.

All forms of private health insurance amount to redistribution of resources from the healthy to the sick. While everyone pays premiums, healthy people go to the doctor less, and so don't actually receive all the benefits they are paying for. Sick people go to the doctor a lot more, and actually consume more services than they pay for. The same could be said for government sponsored insurance, those who pay much of the cost of those services use fewer health resources than they pay for, while their parents and grandparents who receive Medicare use more services than they pay for. The purpose of Medicare, however, is to ensure the elderly and disabled have access to ongoing preventive and primary care in order to prevent unnecessary and excessive hospitalizations, which costs everyone even more.

The United States spends more money on healthcare than any other industrialized country. Figure 10.2 shows that the US spends a total of 17.2% of GDP on health care. This is nearly 50% more than the next most expensive system in Switzerland. The U.S. currently spends $9086 per capita on health care, which is nearly three times the average of all other industrialized nations, who spend an average of $3600 (Squires & Anderson 2015). Based on what we spend, we should expect to have health outcomes significantly better than all those countries that spend less. Unfortunately, that's not the case. According to research conducted by the Commonwealth Fund, of the thirteen countries compared in Fig. 10.2, the United States ranks in the middle of the pack in terms of health care quality. For

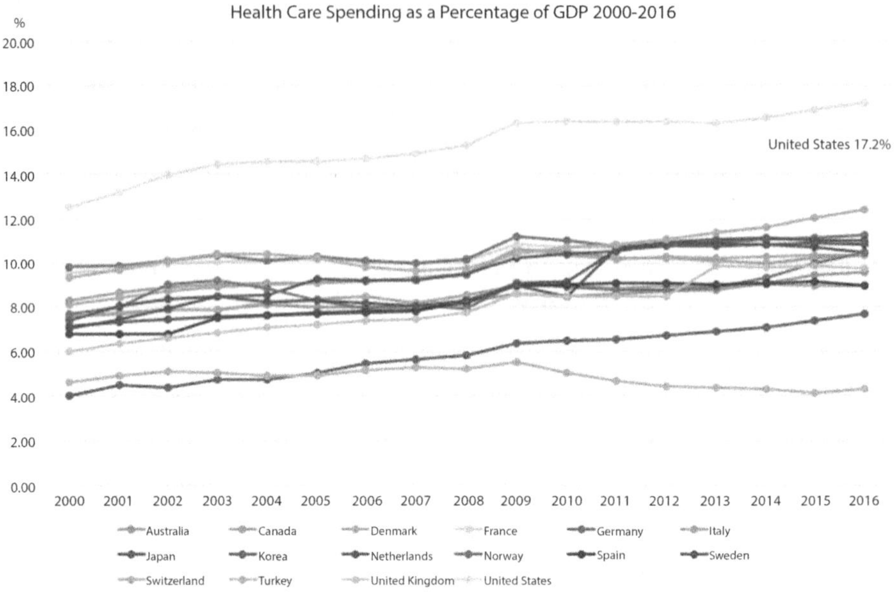

Fig. 10.2 Health Care Spending as Percent of Gross Domestic Product 2000–2016 (Source: OECD (2017), Health expenditure and financing: Health expenditure indicators, OECD Health Statistics (database). https://doi.org/10.1787/data-00349-en (Accessed on 08 September 2017))

example, the U.S. is ranked 6th in survival rates from cancer, and near the bottom, 11th place, on survival rates from ischemic heart disease. Another shortcoming in the U.S. medical care system is uninsurance. Although just over 90% of Americans currently have health insurance coverage, we are still away from the kind of universal coverage enjoyed by nearly all other industrialized nations.

In addition to requiring individuals to purchase health coverage (the mandate) and expanding Medicaid, the Affordable Care Act is also changing the way health care delivery is organized. The creation of Accountable Care Organizations (ACOs) was intended to address the problem of high cost while at the same time improve quality of care. They are expected to do this by requiring health care providers in hopsitals, doctors offices, and health insurers to work together to manage their patients' care. Specifically, rather than simply receiving government payments for services provided, physicians, hospitals, and health insurance companies must show that they are providing appropriate preventive care, are reducing emergency room and hospital visits, and avoiding unecessary tests and treatement. The rules are designed to decrease costs by reducing unecessary care and improve quality by emphasizing prevention so that people stay healthy in the first place. The number of ACOs have grown dramatically, and there are currently more than 838 ACOs in the U.S. caring for more than 6 million Medicare beneficiaries (Muhlestein and McLellan 2016).

So why is healthcare so expensive in this country? According to Dr. David Cutler (2013) there are three main reasons. The first is that administrative costs in the U.S. are twice as high as other countries. For example, about 25% of health care costs are for administration, like patient billing services. This is much higher than Canada, whose administrative costs are only 10–15% of expenditures. The second reason costs are so high is that the prices of all health care services and goods are much higher: not only for drugs, which are much costlier in the U.S. than anywhere else, but doctors get paid more for the same services too. Finally, Americans use more care. Not necessarily primary care visits, which are lower in the U.S. than many other countries, but when someone has a heart attack, for example, they would receive many more services, including open-heart surgery, than they would in other countries. These extra services, however, do not appear to improve health outcomes since outcomes in other countries are equal to or better than the U.S. Since doctors get paid more to do more, the financial incentives are to provide more care whether needed or not. Although it is too soon to understand what impacts ACOs will have on cost and quality, early results suggest that it is doing both (Bodenheimer and Grumbach 2016).

Taken together, the major provisions of the Affordable Care Act including the individual mandate, the expansion of Medicaid, and the establishment of health insurance marketplaces have increased insurance coverage in the U.S. As Fig. 10.3 shows, the rates of uninsurance peaked at 18.2% in 2010, and by 2015 had declined to just over 10% of the adult population. One of the main reasons that there are still more than 28 million uninsured people is that many low income families report that health insurance cost too much, in fact nearly half of all uninsured families recently surveyed suggest that cost was the reason they remain uninsured (Kaiser 2016). Many of the uninsured are people who work in jobs that don't provide coverage, and/or live in states that elected not to expand their Medicaid programs making the cost of coverage out of reach.

10.3.3 Health Care Disparities

Health care is not distributed equally in this country. Racial and ethnic minorities, and people with less education and lower incomes are more likely to be uninsured, have worse access to care, and lower quality of care. As shown in Table 10.2, all minority groups are more likely to be without health insurance compared to Whites. This is a result of a number of factors including an increased likelihood of living in poverty, being unemployed, or being less likely to work in jobs that provide health coverage. Unless insurance coverage is obtained through an employer, the high costs of premiums prevent low income groups from obtaining insurance. Hispanic populations have the worst access due to working in industries that don't provide coverage, along with immigration status (Table 10.2).

Due to the high cost of medical services, access to health care is heavily dependent on health insurance coverage. And the same vulnerable groups that experience

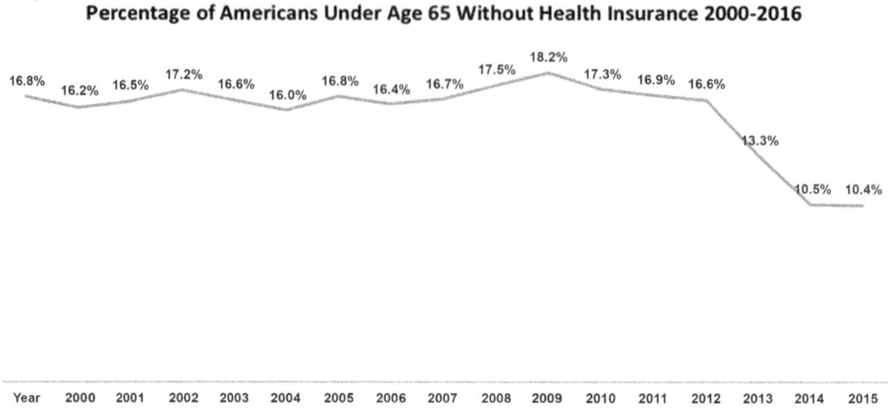

Fig. 10.3 Uninsured rate of non-elderly Americans (Source: Clarke TC, Norris T, Schiller JS. Early release of selected estimates based on data from 2016 National Health Interview Survey. NCHS. May 2017. Available from http://www.cdc.gov/nchs/nhis.htm)

poor access to insurance have much worse access to health care as a result. The uninsured, especially low income and minority groups, are less likely to have a usual source of care, and are more likely to report that they had to delay or forego care. In fact Blacks (21%) and Hispanics (24%) are nearly twice as likely as Whites (14%) to report not receiving needed care (Ubri and Artiga 2016). Among the uninsured with low incomes, more than 75% report being unable to get medical care, dental care, or prescription medications because of the cost (AHRQ 2014).

In addition to high cost, another explanations for poor access to care among vulnerable populations is the geographic distribution of health care resources. For example, for people in rural areas, who also have less education and limited economic resources not only struggle to pay for needed care, but there are also limited doctors and hospitals in rural area that adds significant transportation burden to receiving care (Douthit et al. 2015). Similarly, in poor urban areas characterized by high rates of segregation and concentrated poverty, there are also fewer health care resources including physicians, hospitals and primary care clinics (Kaplan et al. 2015).

Financial and geographic barriers result in reduced access to health care for racial and ethnic minorities and people with low incomes. In turn, reduced access to care results in poor health outcomes. For example, even though African American women have lower rates of breast cancer than white women, because they lack access to care they are more likely to be diagnosed at a later stage and are more likely to die from breast cancer. In fact, uninsured women of all races are significantly more likely than insured women to delay seeing care for breast cancer and have higher mortality rates as a result (Niu et al. 2013). Similarly, rates of death for asthma are much higher among African Americans and Native Americans. Asthma is a treatable disease and only about 1/100,000 whites dies from asthma. The rates of death are twice as high for Native Americans and three times as high for African

Table 10.2 Number and percentage of adults age 18–64 years without health insurance

Number and percentage of adults aged 18–64 years without health insurance, by poverty status and race/ethnicity — National Health Interview Survey, United States, 2010

Characteristic	No.	(% of total)	% without health insurance
Poverty status[a]			
Poor	11,078,526	(30.8)	41.2
Near poor	18,246,425	(50.7)	34.2
Nonpoor	6,641,720	(18.5)	8.1
Total	35,966,671[c]	(100.0)	–
Race/Ethnicity			
Hispanic[b]	11,957,253	(29.3)	41.0
White, non-Hispanic	20,130,159	(49.5)	16.1
Black, non-Hispanic	6,097,277	(15.0)	26.2
American Indian/Alaska Native	363,140	(0.9)	33.5
Asian/Pacific Islander	1,575,972	(3.9)	17.3
Other, non-Hispanic and multiple race	560,459	(1.4)	21.5
Total	40,684,260[c]	(100.0)	–

Source: MMWR November 22, 2013 vol 62 no. 3

[a]Poor = ≤1.0 time the federal poverty level (FPL), near poor = 1.0 2.9 times FPL, and non-poor = ≥3.0 times FPL. FPL was based on U.S. Census Bureau poverty thresholds, available at http://www.census.gov/hhes/www/poverty/html

[b]Persons of hispanic ethnicity might be of any race or combination of races

[c]Totals are different because of unknown poverty status

Americans. Because health insurance means having a regular health care provider, getting routing care, and care for chronic conditions, people with health insurance are less likely to die. Because lack of health insurance coverage has such a strong effect on access to care, more than 44,000 deaths per year for treatable conditions are attributable to lack of health insurance (Wilper et al. 2009).

In addition to poor health care access, vulnerable populations also often face significant barriers in quality of care received. Health care disparities are a result three factors: patient factors, provider factors, and system factors. Among the most important patient factors that lead to disparities in care is patient trust. In particular, there is a legacy of mistrust of health care providers and hospitals among African Americans as a legacy of Tuskegee experiment (see Chap. 6). Ongoing discrimination, however, is also an important factor. Recent research shows that at least 30% of African American report that discrimination is common in doctors' offices, compared to only 7% of White patients (Johnson et al. 2012). African Americans are also much more likely to report being dissatisfied with the care they received, than White patients. This lack of trust, poor communication, and less satisfaction with care leads to poor management of chronic diseases like high blood pressure and diabetes, and leads to avoidable emergency room visits and hospitalizations as a result.

Vulnerable subgroups including racial and ethnic minorities as patients with less income and education are treated differently by physicians. Implicit bias refers to unconscious negative attitudes held by people about racial minorities, and other marginalized groups. Research has shown that like most people, doctors also have implicit bias as a result of being exposed to negative messages about minorities. The mass media, for example, more often depicts African Americans as criminals (See Chap. 7). While implicit bias is a problem in society, it is especially problematic in health care. This is because doctors are required to make important decisions in the context of a short office visit, with limited time to get to know the patient as a person. Faced with the need to make decisions with limited time and information, physicians are affected by implicit bias and thus are more likely to apply stereotypes. One way this plays out is that doctors are less likely to prescribe more aggressive treatment for African Americans than they do for their White patients because they believe that African Americans are less likely to be compliant, or be able to follow complicated treatment regimens (Green et al. 2012). Implicit bias has been shown to affect the care of low income patients as well in much the same way (Van Ryn and Burke 2000). Doctors assume that they will be less compliant, and less able to follow through with complicated treatment regimens.

Pain control is another area where minorities are treated differently by medical providers because of discrimination. African Americans and Hispanics are less likely to receive pain medication than White patients, even when their medical records show that they have similar injuries (Todd et al. 2012). Not only are they less likely to be prescribed pain medication, but for those who return home with a prescription for pain medication, they might find that their pharmacy does not stock it. Pharmacies in poor and minority neighborhoods are less likely to stock narcotic pain medications (Morrison et al. 2000).

Health care systems are often designed to provide services to White, English-speaking populations, and are not able to provide culturally competent care. Although this is slowly changing, it is still the case that for patients with limited English proficiency (LEP), and thus receiving appropriate health services can be very challenging. As many as half of all patients who need interpretive services in their language do not get it, despite the fact that it is mandated by the federal government. In fact many patients with LEP report worse satisfaction with care, and demonstrate worse outcomes as a result of communication problems (Mosen et al. 2004). As described in Chap. 5, cultural barriers extend beyond language. Muslim women, for example, have reported significant barriers in receiving health care that meets their cultural preference for modesty (Hasnain et al. 2011).

A number of factors affect women's health care. Since women are more likely to use health care, they also have more opportunities to have a bad experience. Although women are more likely to have health insurance, and are more likely to have health care visits, they are also more likely to report delayed or foregone care. This includes physician visits as well as needed prescription medications. Women are also more likely to report difficulty paying for medical bills. Both financial and non-financial barriers are to blame. Women are more likely to live in poverty, so even with insurance, out-of-pocket costs are more likely to present a barrier for women than for men. But non-financial barriers are important too, since women roles in society still require that they spend a great deal of time taking care of others, they are often unable to devote adequate time to taking care of themselves. One of the major reasons women report inability to obtain care is because of the time involved. Stereotypes, too, operate in health care encounters for women, just as it does for other vulnerable populations. For example, despite the fact that both men and women die of similar rates from heart disease, women are treated less aggressively by doctors because there is little recognition that women are at equal risk (Keyhani et al. 2008).

Resources, Links, and Recommended Readings

Conrad, P., & Schneider, J. W. (2010). *Deviance and medicalization: From badness to sickness*. Temple University Press.

Marmot, M. (2004). Status Syndrome. *Significance, 1*(4), 150–154.

Bodenheimer, T., & Grumbach, K. (2012). *Understanding health policy*. McGraw Hill Professional.

The Affordable Care Act website provides up-to-date and relevant data and information about many topics including insurance coverage and research related to the AffordableCareAct.https://aspe.hhs.gov/basic-report/health-insurance-coverage-and-affordable-care-act-september-2015

The National Health Care Quality and Disparities Report includes data and reports on health care access and quality for vulnerable populations in the U.S. https://www.ahrq.gov/research/findings/nhqrdr/nhqdr15/access.html

There are a number of TEDx talks related to health disparities and health care. You can find a list of relevant talks here: https://www.ted.com/topics/health+care

Get a global perspective. The World Health Organization social determinants of health website includes a number of educational articles and videos designed to provide current information about the evidence for disparities, and various countries efforts to combat health inequities. http://www.who.int/social_determinants/en/

The Kaiser Family Foundation provides current and comprehensive information about uninsured populations in the United States. It is an excellent resource for developing a better understanding of the causes and consequences of uninsurance. http://www.kff.org/uninsured/

Activities and Research Examples

Activity 1. Mapping out Medicalization

This is an in-class activity designed to introduce the concept of medicalization, or the process by which human problems become understood, defined and treated as being medical in nature. This activity also provides the opportunity to discuss the avenues by which this process occurs and its social implications. Students respond to multiple prompts by labeling states of affairs as being medical conditions or not. The classroom responses are mapped out on a continuum to visually stimulate and guide discussion about the placement of each state of affairs. This activity engages the entire classroom and requires students to interact directly with their classmates in their discussion of medicalization.

Source: Tom, Joshua C. 2014. "Mapping out Medicalization." Class Activity published in *TRAILS: Teaching Resources and Innovations Library for Sociology*. Washington DC: American Sociological Association. (http://trails.asanet.org).

http://trails.asanet.org/Pages/Resource.aspx?ResourceID=12858

Activity 2. Visit the Southern Poverty Law Center's Teaching Tolerance, Health Disparities website: http://www.tolerance.org/lesson/health-disparities. This website includes a number of activities designed to help explore the causes and consequences of health disparities, and create possible solutions for overcoming them.

Key Terms and Definitions

- **Health** is a state of complete physical, mental and social well-being and not merely the absence of disease or infirmity.
- **Medicine** the social institution responsible for delivering medical care.
  - **Medicalization** refers to the increasing tendency to treat problems previously defined as non-medical, in medical terms. Delivery of health care
  - **Illness experience** is the social process in which a diagnosis or subjective label is applied to someone. That label both affects how others see them, and how they see themselves.
  - **Social epidemiology** is the study of the social and environmental causes and consequences of disease.
- **Health Disparities** inequalities in health that vary by race, ethnicity, social class, and gender.
- **Health Care Disparities** inequalities in the provision of health services that vary by race, ethnicity, social class, and gender.

Study Questions

1. **Describe the positive and negative aspects of medicalization. Be sure to give examples of each.**
2. **Describe racial and ethnic disparities in health care. Which groups are at highest risk for poor access and quality?**

***Example Exam Question**: Which of the following is the most common source of payment for health care in the U.S.?

(a) **Self-pay**
(b) **Individual Private Insurance**
(c) **Employment-based insurance**
(d) **Public Insurance**

The above example is an author created question, please visit https://students-residents.aamc.org/applying-medical-school/article/whats-mcat-exam/ for more information for more information.

References

2014 National Healthcare Quality and Disparities Report. Rockville: Agency for Healthcare Research and Quality; May 2015. AHRQ Pub. No. 15-0007.

Association of American Medical Colleges (AAMC). (2015). *The official guide to the MCAT exam (MCAT2015)* (4th ed.). Washington, DC: The Association of American Medical Colleges.

Berwick, D. M., & Hackbarth, A. D. (2012). Eliminating waste in US health care. *Jama, 307*(14), 1513–1516.

Bodenheimer, T. S., & Grumbach, K. (2016). *Understanding health policy: A clinical approach* (5th ed.). New York: McGraw-Hill Companies, Inc.

Cutler, D. (2013). *Why does health care cost so much in America? Ask Harvard's David Cutler*. http://www.pbs.org/newshour/rundown/why-does-health-care-cost-so-much-in-america-ask-harvards-david-cutler/

Douthit, N., Kiv, S., Dwolatzky, T., & Biswas, S. (2015). Exposing some important barriers to health care access in the rural USA. *Public Health, 129*(6), 611–620.

Grad, F. P. (2002).The Preamble of the Constitution of the World Health Organization, *Bulletin of the World Health Organization, 80*(12), 981. http://www.who.int/bulletin/archives/80(12)981.pdf

Green, A. R., Carney, D. R., Pallin, D. J., Ngo, L. H., Raymond, K. L., Iezzoni, L. I., & Banaji, M. R. (2012). Implicit bias among physicians and its prediction of thrombolysis decisions for Black and White patients. In T. A. LaVeist & L. A. Isaac (Eds.), *Race, ethnicity, and health: A public health reader* (Vol. 32, pp. 569–586). San Francisco, CA: Wiley.

Gruber, J. (2010). *The tax exclusion for employer-sponsored health insurance* (No. w15766). National Bureau of Economic Research.

Hasnain, M., Connell, K. J., Menon, U., & Tranmer, P. A. (2011). Patient-centered care for Muslim women: provider and patient perspectives. *Journal of Women's Health, 20*(1), 73–83.

Johnson, RL, Roter, D, Powe NR, & Cooper LA. (2012). Patient race/ethnicity and quality of patient communication during medical visits. In T. A. LaVeist & L. A. Isaac (Eds.), *Race, ethnicity, and health: A public health reader* (Vol. 32, pp. 569–606). San Francisco, CA: Wiley.

Kaiser Family Foundation. (2016). *Key facts about the uninsured population*. http://kff.org/uninsured/fact-sheet/key-facts-about-the-uninsured-population/

Kaplan, R., Spittel, M., & David, D. (Eds). 2015, July. *Population health: Behavioral and social science insights*. AHRQ Publication No. 15–0002. Rockville: Agency for Healthcare Research and Quality and Office of Behavioral and Social Sciences Research, National Institutes of Health.

Keyhani, S., Scobie, J. V., Hebert, P. L., & McLaughlin, M. A. (2008). Gender disparities in blood pressure control and cardiovascular care in a national sample of ambulatory care visits. *Hypertension, 51*(4), 1149–1155.

Kivimäki, M., & Kawachi, I. (2015). Work stress as a risk factor for cardiovascular disease. *Current Cardiology Reports, 17*(9), 74.

Kurani, N., Ranji, U., Salganicoff, A., & Rae, M. (2017). *Paid family leave and sick days in the U.S.: Findings from the 2016 Kaiser/HRET Employer Health Benefits Survey*. Kaiser Family Foundation http://files.kff.org/attachment/Data-Note-Paid-Family-Leave-and-Sick-Days-in-the-US-Findings-from-the-2016-Kaiser-HRET-Employer-Health-Benefits-Survey

Lauderdale, D. S. (2006). Birth outcomes for Arabic-named women in California before and after September 11. *Demography, 43*(1), 185–201.

Link, B. G., & Phelan, J. (1995). Social conditions as fundamental causes of disease. *Journal of Health and Social Behavior, 36*, 80–94.

Marmot, M. (2004). *The status syndrome: How your social standing affects your health and life expectancy*. London: Bloomsbury.

Morrison, R. S., Wallenstein, S., Natale, D. K., Senzel, R. S., & Huang, L. L. (2000). "We don't carry that"—failure of pharmacies in predominantly nonwhite neighborhoods to stock opioid analgesics. *New England Journal of Medicine, 342*(14), 1023–1026.

Mosen, D. M., Carlson, M. J., Morales, L. S., & Hanes, P. P. (2004). Satisfaction with provider communication among Spanish-speaking Medicaid enrollees. *Ambulatory Pediatrics, 4*(6), 500–504.

Muhlestein, D., & Mclellan, M. (2016). *Accountable care organizations in 2016: Private and public sector growth and dispersion*. Health Affairs Blog April 21st, 2016. http://healthaffairs.org/blog/2016/04/21/accountable-care-organizations-in-2016-private-and-public-sector-growth-and-dispersion/

National Center for Health Statistics. (2014). *Health, United States, 2013: With special feature on prescription drugs*. Hyattsville.

Niu, X., Roche, L. M., Pawlish, K. S., & Henry, K. A. (2013). Cancer survival disparities by health insurance status. *Cancer medicine, 2*(3), 403–411.

Schnittker, J. (2007). Working more and feeling better: women's health, employment, and family life, 1974–2004. *American Sociological Review, 72*(2), 221–238.

Squires, D., & Anderson, C. (2015). US health care from a global perspective: spending, use of services, prices, and health in 13 countries. *The Commonwealth Fund, 15*, 1–16.

Todd, K. H., Deaton, C., D'Adamo, A. P., & Goe, L. (2012). Ethnicity and analgesic practice. In T. A. LaVeist & L. A. Isaac (Eds.), *Race, ethnicity, and health: A public health reader* (Vol. 32, pp. 637–646). Wiley: San Francisco.

Ubri, P., & Artiga, S. (2016). *Disparities in health and health care: Five key questions and answers*. Kaiser family foundation. http://files.kff.org/attachment/Issue-Brief-Disparities-in-Health-and-Health-Care-Five-Key-Questions-and-Answers

Van Ryn, M., & Burke, J. (2000). The effect of patient race and socio-economic status on physicians' perceptions of patients. *Social Science & Medicine, 50*(6), 813–828.

Williams, D. R., Mohammed, S. A., Leavell, J., & Collins, C. (2010). Race, socioeconomic status, and health: Complexities, ongoing challenges, and research opportunities. *Annals of the New York Academy of Sciences, 1186*(1), 69–101.

Wilper, A. P., Woolhandler, S., Lasser, K. E., McCormick, D., Bor, D. H., & Himmelstein, D. U. (2009). Health insurance and mortality in US adults. *American Journal of Public Health, 99*(12), 2289–2295.

Women and Health Care in the Early Years of the ACA: Key Findings from the 2013 Kaiser Women's Health Survey, May 15 2014, Alina Salganicoff.

Zimmerman, E. B., Woolf, S. H., & Haley, A. Search Health Topics Health Care Delivery. (2015). *Understanding the relationship between education and health: A review of the evidence and an examination of community perspectives*. Content last reviewed September 2015. Agency for Healthcare Research and Quality, Rockville. http://www.ahrq.gov/professionals/education/curriculum-tools/population-health/zimmerman.html

CPSIA information can be obtained
at www.ICGtesting.com
Printed in the USA
LVHW080051311218
602233LV00012B/360/P

9 783319 649481